THE MUSCLE
FITNESS

D1386907

THE
MUSCLE FITNESS
BOOK

Francine St George

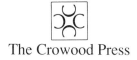

The Crowood Press

ACKNOWLEDGEMENTS

The completion of this book would not have been possible without the continual support of my work colleagues, who permitted me time between a busy schedule of clinical work, travel and lecturing, to bring this book together. Particular thanks go to Kerry Coffey, Gary Egger and Robyn Gant for their assistance with editing; to Steve Keen for his computer skills, and to Monika Durach, Carol Knight and my sister Dale McCosker, for their typing expertise.

A very special thanks goes to Jenny Hall for her invaluable role in the preparation of the original artwork and the manuscript.

My final thanks go to my patients, whose constant questioning made me realise I needed to write this book, and last but not least, to my publisher, Kirsty Melville, and my editors, Ariana Klepac and Julia Cain, at Simon & Schuster, for their patience and professionalism.

THE MUSCLE FITNESS BOOK
First published in Australasia in 1989 by
Simon & Schuster Australia
7 Grosvenor Place, Brookvale NSW 2100

A division of Gulf + Western

© Francine St George, 1989

Published in 1990 by
The Crowood Press
Gipsy Lane, Swindon
Wiltshire SN2 6DQ

British Library Cataloguing in Publication Data

St George, Francine
    The muscle fitness book.
    1. Physical fitness
    I. Title
    613.7
ISBN 1-85223-577-2

Designed by Helen Semmler
Illustrations by Heather Strahan
Index by Jill Matthews Hi Tech Editing
Typeset in Hong Kong by Best-set in Century
Printed in England by Clays Ltd., St. Ives plc

CONTENTS

FOREWORD

The Muscle Fitness Book provides practical and comprehensive guide-lines for safe and sensible exercise programmes. It will appeal to a wide range of active people from the beginner setting out on a fitness programme, to the experienced sportsperson seeking a more specific type of training. A particular theme throughout the book is one of safe exercise and quality of movement and there is an awareness of the potential dangers of incorrect or inappropriate exercise which may cause injury.

The early part of the book outlines the relevant theory based on the major systems of the body, but naturally concentrates on the musculoskeletal system, in an encouraging and understandable way. This is followed by a substantial practical section which includes a wealth of well-chosen exercises for stretching, strengthening and daily routines. The detailed exercise programmes, which include exercises which are not recommended and give safe alternatives, are supported, as is the case throughout the book, with clear, precise diagrams and illustrations. This leads into a helpful section for particularly important groups in the community ranging from young children, to people with back problems, to the over 50s. The sportsperson is well catered for with specific exercise programmes across a range of popular sports. In typically realistic fashion the conclusion of the book outlines what to do in the event of injury and provides a clear outline of common injuries with practical suggestions for self-help and treatment.

Francine St George is a well-known physiotherapist from Sydney, Australia, who has had ten years of intensive clinical experience as well as lecturing on exercise and fitness in Australia and overseas. Most importantly she has had regular contact with sport through her private practices in Sydney and through lecturing to coaches, fitness advisers, physiotherapists and fitness leaders in the community. She has combined her professional expertise as a physiotherapist with a working knowledge of sport to produce a valuable practical handbook on exercise and fitness for all types of participant.

Rex Hazeldine
Director of Exercise Physiology
British Olympic Medical Centre

INTRODUCTION

Keeping fit should be fun. For the converted and addicted it usually is, but for the injured it is not. 'Rest' is not a fun word.

From my clinical experience as a physiotherapist, it always intrigues me that whatever the current fitness craze, no matter what sport one plays, the type of injuries one sustains are usually predictable. If you run you suffer runner's knee; if you swim it is swimmer's shoulder; or if you play tennis or golf you are entitled to have an elbow problem. More recently with the craze in aerobic dance, shin splints and back or hip problems have become the most common complaints.

It seems to me, therefore, that something is wrong. If we know so well what problem a person will get from playing a particular sport, why is all the stretching and intensive training people are doing for their sport not preventing it? Are they even doing too much stretching and creating more problems? One *can* overstretch.

The answer seems to me that we are not seeking far enough back into the process that has eventually led to these injuries. Why are some people so vulnerable to injury and others not? Why do some people train and never get injured while others copy their programmes and are forced to retire from sport? With time and experience it soon becomes obvious that the key factor which is being overlooked is that of posture.

Posture, particularly poor posture, appears to be directly related to the incidence of injury one suffers. The worse the posture the higher the incidence of injury. Therefore, it seems necessary to establish if a person is really suited to a particular sport, and if they have taken the necessary measures and precautions to enable their body to start their chosen activity. That is, have they assessed their posture to identify where they are predisposed to injury?

When patients ask me where they can find, in book form, the postural corrective exercises they are taught during treatment, I have nowhere to refer them. Either the available books are too technical and detailed or they are too simple. *The Muscle Fitness Book* has been written to meet these needs.

The book is designed to be a comprehensive and practical guide for the person wanting to become fit, as well as for the individual who is already engaged in a fitness programme but who wishes to prevent any occurrence or recurrence of an injury. In addition it is for the health professional who wants ideas about exercises suitable for both a wide variety of sports and postural correction. This book aims to provide these ideas.

The Muscle Fitness Book is divided into three parts. The first reviews the major systems of the body but focuses on the musculoskeletal system. How to go about taking up a fitness programme but not become disillusioned by injury, is the concern of the opening chapters. Questions commonly asked regarding muscle fitness are also answered, such as: how muscles work, why we need to stretch, how we can be careful we do not overstretch, and so on. There are many facts and fallacies published on the topic of exercise and muscle fitness — almost daily. *The Muscle Fitness Book* attempts to separate truth from fiction.

The second part of the book comprises the practical component. Stretching, basic strengthening and mobility exercises are shown for each part of the body in addition to daily routines for groups with special needs such as the traveller, desk worker, musician and hypermobile (overflexible). Basic routines for the most popular sports and activities complete this section. For each sport a diagram is provided which clearly shows the areas most vulnerable to injury. The most important issues regarding each sport are discussed.

Finally, in Part 3, who one can turn to when injuries are sustained and basic self-help measures are suggested. Have you ever had an injury and no matter who you turned to (friend, colleague or health professional), they all had a different solution for you on how you could help it heal? This section tries to clarify this often very confusing area.

The most important feature of *The Muscle Fitness Book* is that it is not just another sports injury book. It is a book written to assist you to understand why injuries even happen. Many of the exercises in this book will initially appear to conflict with what you may have previously been told you should not do. This is because every exercise in this book is safe as long as it is performed with care and not done at high speed, in an out-of-control manner, as often happens in fitness classes. This can either directly or indirectly lead to injury. No two persons' bodies are the same. We all require a slightly different exercise pro- gramme. *The Muscle Fitness Book* will enable everyone to design an exercise programme which suits their specific needs.

All exercises should be performed with quality movements and *should not cause pain*. *The Muscle Fitness Book* is written for those who want to improve the efficiency and quality of how their bodies move, both on an everyday basis, and for their sport.

HOW TO USE MUSCLE FITNESS

The ideal way to achieve muscle fitness is to review the basic theory in Part 1 of the book and design your own programme for correcting your posture. Then you should combine this routine with those exercises shown for your specific sport. These exercises are most important prior to your activity but they may also be performed afterwards, as well as in between exercise sessions. If any exercise is unclear, always consult a sports specialist to ensure you are not doing it incorrectly. It is always wiser to be overcautious than undercautious when it comes to keeping our muscles fit.

Just remember — if you can predict injury you can prevent injury, so have lots of fun but always be careful.

PART 1 — THE BODY, MUSCLES AND EXERCISE

1 — HOW THE BODY WORKS

Before we start analysing muscles and discussing muscle fitness we need to understand what structures the body comprises. This section will review the major systems of the body. These include the cardiovascular, respiratory, gastrointestinal, lymphatic, nervous and the craniosacral and musculoskeletal systems. The focus in the second half of this chapter will be on the musculoskeletal system as this is the most important system to understand to achieve muscle fitness. Later on in Chapter 4 we will discuss the cardiovascular system in more detail when we are reviewing exercise, sport and muscles.

THE MAJOR SYSTEMS OF THE BODY

The basic unit of the body is the cell which exists in all shapes and sizes. It is within the protoplasm, or jelly-like substance of the cell, that complex biochemical changes occur, creating the processes of life as we know them.

Groups of cells which perform similar functions are referred to as tissue. Examples of tissue are muscles, nerves and the connective tissue that separates and supports these structures. These tissues in turn form organs such as the heart, lungs, glands, the skeleton and the skin. Organs and tissue with similar functions comprise the body's main systems.

To enable all the structures of the body to function, they receive oxygen carried in the blood through arteries from the heart, and the veins which pump the used blood back to the heart. This system of blood flow is called the *cardiovascular system*. Your pulse rate (the rhythmic pumping of the arteries) is an indication of how efficient your heart is. For normal healthy individuals, the slower your pulse rate the fitter you are.

The *respiratory system* refers to the lungs and airways. We breathe in oxygen and exhale carbon dioxide. (Plants alternatively utilise carbon dioxide to stay alive and exhale oxygen.) When resting, we breathe air in at eight to twelve breaths per minute. This air which is rich in oxygen is then taken by the heart and pumped throughout the body in the blood.

The *gastrointestinal system* includes all the structures involved in the digestion of food. The stomach, small and large intestines, pancreas and liver are all part of this system. These organs are often referred to as viscera.

The *lymphatic system* is the system responsible for fighting infection and comprises very thin vessels which carry a clearish fluid. Nodules called lymph nodes may be found at certain places, mainly in the arm-pit or the groin area. Infection causes these to enlarge.

Another system, the *nervous system*, is that system comprising the brain, spinal cord and nerves. The latter carry messages to the muscles, organs and viscera. Nerves emerge from in between each vertebra from the spinal cord which is a direct extension of the brain.

The *craniosacral system* is a less well known system. This system refers to the cranium (the skull) and how it is linked up with the sacrum (the base of the spine). Fluid flows up and down the spinal canals and cushions the brain within the skull. This fluid is called the cerebrospinal fluid and is produced in the brain. It is pumped up and down the spine at a rate of six to twelve beats, or cycles, per minute. This pulse is less easily detectable by the individual, but can be palpated anywhere in the body by a skilled craniosacral therapist.

All these systems work together to keep our body functioning as an efficient machine. No one system can go wrong without having an effect elsewhere in the body, either directly or indirectly, in the short or long term. It is almost as if a chain reaction occurs. For this reason the body can be viewed as a closed 'kinetic' system, that is, it is continually changing, adapting and altering due to both intrinsic (the body's actual systems) and extrinsic (outer environmental) forces.

In *The Muscle Fitness Book* we will be primarily concerned with the *musculo-skeletal system*, our priority being the muscles. As we learn about them it will soon become clear how something as simple as a sprained ankle, which may force our body to compensate if we have been limping, may be affecting the spine and neck and even producing headaches because of tight neck muscles. They may sound remotely connected, yet this is how complex our body is. So often our body tells us it needs attention, yet we ignore it. Pain is Nature's way of telling us something is wrong, but for some strange reason we have been conditioned to believe we must ignore and cope with our aches and pains. Worse still, we may be told they are part and parcel of getting old. How depressing to be told you cannot change your body just because you are beyond a certain age! Such comments are pure fallacy. Adequate and appropriate exercise, good nutrition and a positive mental attitude can all counteract this supposed ageing effect which is considered inevitable. *The Muscle Fitness Book* shows us how to do this safely and effectively.

THE MUSCULOSKELETAL SYSTEM

The skeleton

Basically, the body is a bundle of bones; 226 altogether. Bones are important because they provide attachment for our muscles and also a stable structure for supporting our organs as well as our muscles. The skeleton consists of a group of long bones, in the arms and legs, for movement; shorter and smaller bones, in the hands and feet, for manoeuvrability; the vertebrae of the back and the bones of the pelvis which provide support; and lastly the rib cage and the skull to protect the body's vital organs.

Bones are linked together in various ways at the joints. Ball and socket (for example, the shoulder and hip), and hinge (the knee), are the major types of joints. Other joints are sliding joints (the wrist and ankle), pivot (the first cervical vertebra at the base of the skull which rotates around the second cervical vertebra) and the vertebral joints which connect the vertebrae of the spine. Most joint surfaces in our limbs are protected by cartilage and fluid. These are called synovial joints. In the spine, the vertebrae are cushioned and separated by cartilaginous discs. These provide shock absorption for the spine.

All joints have an *active* range of movement made possible by the muscles which contract around the joint, and a *passive* range of movement. Range of movement simply refers to how far we can move a joint. Active range of movement is how far we, ourselves, can move a joint consciously by contracting our muscles, such as when raising our arms above our heads. Passive range of movement means the extra movement that takes place in a joint that the individual cannot consciously control, but which can be achieved by a therapist. Techniques such as mobilisation and manipulation, performed by trained health professionals, can be used to achieve passive range of movement of joints. Injury to muscles usually results in stiffness due to loss of, or reduced, passive joint range in underlying joints. Until both active and passive range of movement are gained, stiffness in a joint may be felt, or recurrence of an injury may occur.

All joints are stabilised by the ligaments which act like strong elastic bands. Figure 1.1 shows the major bones in our skeletal system.

The muscles

Obviously it is impossible to review all the 450 muscles in the body in a book of this size. Figure 1.2, however, shows the most important muscles. This will make it clearer when we are discussing the exercises for specific areas of the body.

In most parts of the body there are layers of muscles. Larger muscles tend to be towards the surface while the smaller muscles tend to be found in the deeper layers, providing stability for joints and for further refining gross (larger) movements. For example, the short deep muscles in the back provide stability between each vertebra when we bend forwards to lift heavy objects, while the larger, more superficial muscles contract through a much greater range. When exercising, it is important to stretch and strengthen all muscles through their full range, as daily activities rarely do this and adaptive shortening of the deeper muscles can occur. This in turn can cause the stiffness we start to feel as we age. Regular stretching, strengthening and improving our posture can minimise this effect.

Figure 1.2 shows most of the superficial muscles as well as some of the more pertinent muscles in the deeper layers. It will be important to check with these diagrams when you are doing the exercises for your particular sport, so you can work on the muscles predisposed to injury, shown on the sports diagrams in Chapter 8.

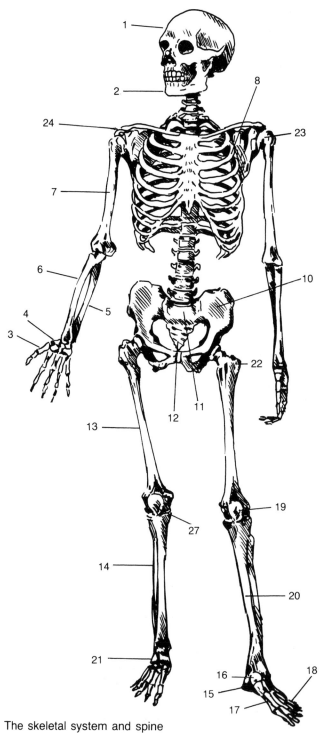

Figure 1.1   The skeletal system and spine

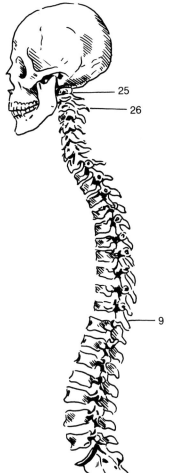

- 25
- 26
- 9

1. Skull
2. Mandible (the lower jaw)
3. Metacarpal bones
4. Carpal bones
5. Ulnar
6. Radius
7. Humerus
8. The ribs
9. The vertebral column
10. Ilium (hip)
11. Sacrum
12. Coccyx
13. Femur
14. Fibula
15. Calcaneum
16. Talus
17. Metatarsal bones
18. The phalanges
19. Patella (knee-cap)
20. Tibia
21. Lateral malleolus
22. Greater trochanter
23. Glenohumeral: the shoulder joint; a ball and socket joint
24. Acromioclavicular joint
25. Atlas
26. Axis
27. Tibiofemoral joint: the knee joint, a hinge joint

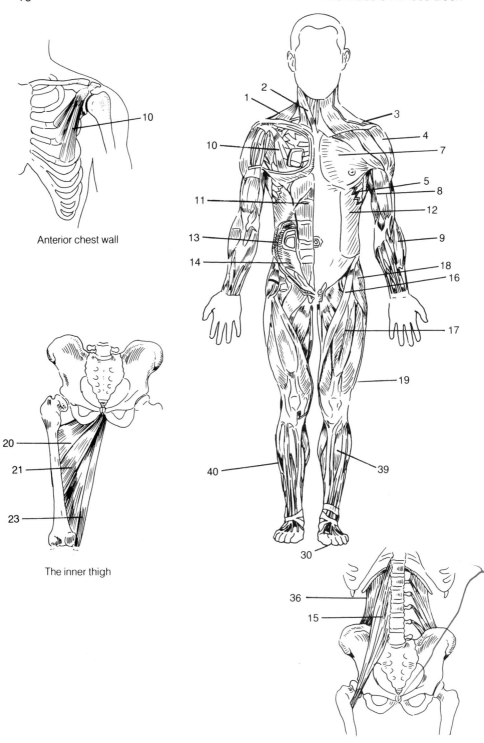

Anterior chest wall

The inner thigh

Deeper muscles of the hip and back

Figure 1.2   Anatomy review

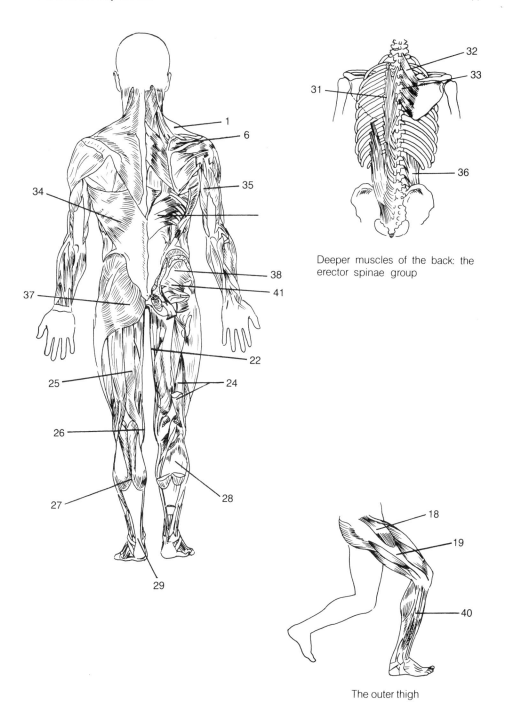

Deeper muscles of the back: the erector spinae group

The outer thigh

See the following pages for key to numbers

Figure 1.2

1. Trapezius — Has four parts. The upper fibres elevate the shoulder, while the lower fibres raise and draw the shoulder blades together. When the lower fibres are weak, this increases the rounded shoulder look that results with poor posture.

2. Sternocleidomastoid — Rotates and side flexes the head to the opposite side.

3. Levator scapulae — Elevates the shoulder blade (for example, when we shrug our shoulders).

4. Deltoid — Has three parts. This muscle contributes to all movements of the upper arm. Anterior fibres assist with flexion, middle fibres with abduction and the posterior fibres with extension.

5. Serratus anterior — This muscle originates from the outer surface of the ribs and inserts onto the medial border of the scapula. It abducts the scapula and when it is weak, a winged effect of the scapula is present.

6. Supraspinatus — A small muscle which initiates abduction of the shoulder joint.

7. Pectoralis major — Adducts the arm and rotates it inwards as is usually seen in people with rounded shoulders.

8. Biceps — Has two parts which help to bend and supinate the elbow. It is used when you pick something up in your hand and turn it over to look at it.

9. Brachioradialis — Bends the elbow, pronates and supinates the forearm, depending on the starting position. It usually is the muscle affected with 'tennis elbow'.

10. Pectoralis minor — Depresses the shoulder blade and rotates the head of the humerus forwards and downwards. If it is tight, an excessive hollow is seen under the clavicle.

11. Rectus abdominis — The abdominal muscle which runs from the sternum down to the pubic bone. It flexes the trunk and is used when performing a sit-up for the first 30 degrees that the head and shoulders are raised. When the head and neck are in a thrust forward position, the rectus becomes shortened.

12. External oblique — Turns the trunk at an angle and is used when performing an oblique sit-up. Becomes weakened and overstretched when a lordotic posture is adopted. Because of where it inserts, it is often referred to as the lower abdominal muscle.

13. Internal oblique — Lies under the external oblique. External and internal oblique work together. It also assists the rectus abdominus in flexing the trunk, especially when performing upper abdominal work (such as in bent-leg sit-ups).

14. Transverse abdominis — Pulls the abdomen in. If the abdominal muscles protrude when you are performing a sit-up, then this muscle is not working effectively.

15. Iliopsoas — Flexes the hip and rotates the leg outwards. When tight and shortened, the spine becomes excessively lordosed.

16. Sartorius — This is often called the 'tailor's muscle'. It is the longest muscle in the body. It flexes, abducts, and rotates the hip outwards. At the knee joint, it bends and rotates the knee inwards.

17. Quadriceps — Has four parts, (a) Rectus femoris flexes the hip and extends the knee while (b) vastis lateralis, (c) vastis intermedialis and (d) vastis medialis extend the knee only. Pain under the knee-cap, often called runner's knee, is caused by faulty biomechanics where three of the quadriceps (which pull the knee-cap laterally), become too strong for the inside quadricep (vastis medialis). Strengthening of this muscle can often rectify this complaint.

18. Tensor fascia latae — Abducts the hip, internally rotates the femur and combined with the iliotibial band, externally rotates the tibia. It assists the lateral stability of the knee.

19. Iliotibial band — A fibrous extension of the tensor fascia latae that inserts in the lateral side of the knee and internally rotates the femur. If, when you stand, your femurs are rotated inwards, it may be due to tightness of this muscle as well as the adductors.

20. Adductor brevis — Is the shorter adductor which adducts the hip and turns the leg inwards.

21. Adductor longus — Long adductor which swings the leg towards the mid-line. It inserts half-way down the femur. If it is tight a marked curvature of the muscle on the inside of the thigh becomes apparent.

22. Gracilis — This is along the slender inside thigh muscle. It is more fibritic than the other adductors. It adducts the hip, bends the knee and turns the knee inwards.

23. Adductor magnus — Is the largest adductor muscle. It adducts the hip, and can also rotate it inwards. Stretching and strengthening of this adductor can help prevent groin injuries that so often occur in contact sports such as soccer and rugby.

24. Biceps femoris — Has two parts. Both are part of the hamstring group. Its action is to extend the hip, flex the knee and turn the knee outwards.

25. Semimembranosus and 26. Semitendinosus — These are the second part of the hamstring group. They straighten the hip, bend the knee and turn it inwards.

27. Gastrocnemius — This muscle makes up two-thirds of the calf muscle. It bends the knee, and plantarflexes the ankle. It is very important for running and jumping activities.

28. Soleus — This is the flat muscle which acts only on the ankle joint (not the knee). It is the other one-third of the calf muscle group. It plantarflexes the ankle.

29. Achilles tendon — The gastrocnemius and soleus muscles together form this tendon which inserts into the heel bone, the calcaneum. Faulty foot mechanics, such as flat feet, can cause pain in this tendon.

30. Intrinsic foot muscles — There are a number of muscles which run within the foot itself. They increase the arch of the foot and provide mobility and flexibility of the rear, mid- and forefoot. The intrinsics include the short toe plantarflexors, adductors and abductors of the toes, and the lumbricals which run between the toes.

31. Erector spinae group — This group consists of muscles of differing lengths which all work as a unit, although some can work in isolation. Together they extend the side and flex and rotate the trunk. Together they are often called the back extensors.

32. Rhomboids minor — This muscle adducts and rotates the shoulder blade inwards. It also helps to keep the shoulder blades flat onto the posterior rib cage.

33. Rhomboids major — This muscle works in combination with rhomboids minor to keep the shoulder blades flat. In sedentary occupations it can get very overstretched because of poor posture.

34. Latissimus dorsi — This is a broad back muscle that forms the back wall of the armpit and pulls the arm behind the back and rotates it inwards. It is very overdeveloped and strong in swimmers.

35. Triceps — Has three parts. It extends the elbow after it has been bent (flexed by the biceps).

36. Quadratus lumborum — This muscle is the most important sideways trunk flexor when movement occurs at the lumbar spine.

37. Gluteus maximus — This is the large buttock muscle. It extends and adducts the hip and turns the thigh outwards.

38. Gluteus medius — Primarily an abductor and internal rotator of the hip.

39. Tibialis anterior — The muscle on the front of the shin bone that dorsiflexes and supinates the foot.

40. Peroneals — Has two major parts, (a) peroneus longus and (b) peroneus brevis, both dorsiflex and pronate the ankle. Peroneus longus builds up the arch of the foot.

41. Piriformis — Lies deep next to the gluteus maximus. When it is tight, an outwardly turned foot will be seen as this is its prime role (to externally rotate the hip). It is assisted in this action by five other external rotators.

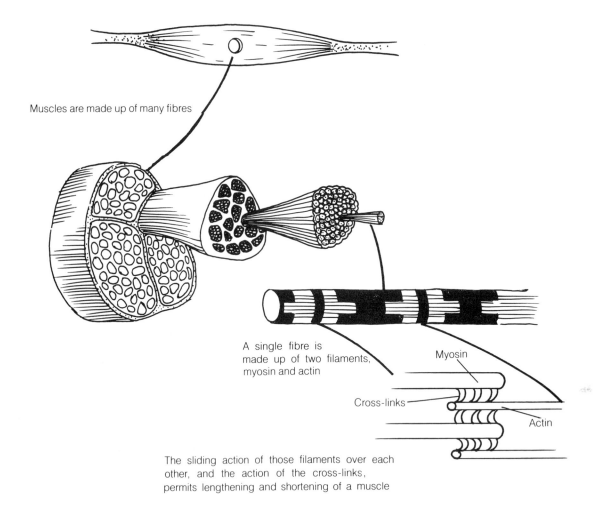

Muscles are made up of many fibres

A single fibre is made up of two filaments, myosin and actin

Myosin

Cross-links

Actin

The sliding action of those filaments over each other, and the action of the cross-links, permits lengthening and shortening of a muscle

1.3   The structure of muscle

Types of muscles

A muscle is an elastic structure that supports, protects and permits movement in the body. Muscles may differ in length, shape, and size. Within our body they comprise at least 40 per cent of our body weight. The human body has over 450 muscles. These muscles are divided into three basic types, dependent on their function, called skeletal, smooth and cardiac muscles.

Skeletal muscles are those such as arm, leg and back muscles. These muscles are associated with voluntary movement of the body (controlled by us at will). If we wish to move our leg or foot, for example, electrical impulses are sent from the brain via the nerves, and these activate the relevant muscle.

Smooth muscles are found in the stomach and arteries and are associated with involuntary movement. These muscles work continuously even when we are asleep. The smooth muscles permit the arteries to pump the blood flow away from the heart and the veins, also under involuntary control, pump the used blood back.

Cardiac muscles are those found in and around the heart. These are also associated with involuntary movement and work continuously to keep the heart pumping.

The importance of muscles

Muscles cover ligaments, bones and joints and permit movement by shortening or contracting to pull our bones into motion. They also provide shape to our skeletal frame. In any sporting activity hundreds of muscles are playing their part. Smooth and cardiac muscles ensure the flow of oxygenated blood around the body to provide nutrients to the working or skeletal muscles, which are able to move the various parts of the body required for any particular sport.

Structure of muscle

All muscles are made up of smaller filaments called myofibrils. On a microscopic level some of these filaments are thick and some thin. The former are called actin and the latter myosin filaments. Figure 1.3 illustrates the relative size of these filaments in relation to the muscle. A bridging, locking mechanism, which prevents the filaments from disengaging once they get to a certain length, permits motion of each muscle within a certain range.

Muscle shape

Skeletal muscles are usually one of three different shapes. These are: unipennate, such as the rectus femoris (in the thigh); bipennate, such as the biceps (in the upper arm); and multipennate, for example the deltoid (at the top of the shoulder). See Figure 1.4.

Muscle action

The action a muscle performs is determined by a number of factors. The most

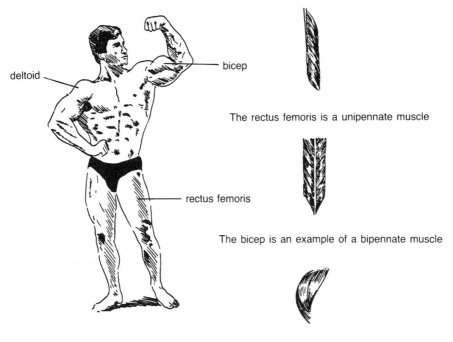

deltoid

bicep

The rectus femoris is a unipennate muscle

rectus femoris

The bicep is an example of a bipennate muscle

The deltoid is a multipennate muscle

1.4   Shapes of muscle

important of these is where the muscle starts, called its origin, and where it finishes or attaches to the bone, called its insertion. The length of the muscle, what type of joint it overlies and in what direction its fibres run (that is, its shape — see Figure 1.4) determine the specific action a muscle performs. Muscles may overlie one, two or a number of joints, permitting different actions for the one muscle.

When two ends of a muscle are brought closer together this is called a concentric contraction. When the two ends move apart this is called an eccentric contraction. An isometric contraction is when the length of a muscle does not alter but is placed against a resistance, for example, the forearm muscles in an arm wrestle.

Muscles may work as an individual unit or with other surrounding muscles to perform a particular movement. The main muscle used to move a joint is called the agonist or prime mover. Muscles assisting the action are called synergists. Other muscles may be required to stabilise to permit a movement. These are called fixators. Muscles that need to relax and lengthen to permit the movement are called the antagonists. Smooth sporting action may become inhibited if agonist/antagonist imbalance exists. For example, tight back extensors (muscles that run the length of the spine) may inhibit the abdominal or stomach muscles from contracting effectively when doing a sit-up — often called an abdominal crunch. A slight tremor, or quivering of the stomach muscles can be observed when performing a sit-up, if these back muscles are tight.

MOVEMENT TERMS AND ANATOMICAL POSITIONS

The terms given to the way muscles move the body are defined and then clarified in reference to the upper limb. These terms can be applied to movement of all body parts.

Flexion A movement which makes the angle between two bones at their joint smaller, for example, when the arm is moved forward and up in relation to the body from the shoulder joint.

Extension This is the opposite action to flexion. It occurs when the arm is moved behind and backwards from the body or when the elbow is straightened from a bent (flexed) position.

Supination Where the sole of the foot or hand is turned inward and upward, for example, a foot with a high arch is usually supinated.

Pronation Where the sole of the foot or hand is turned inward, for example, excessive pronation is observed when the arch of the foot is collapsed to ground level.

Inversion When the forefoot is turned inwards.

Eversion When the forefoot is turned outwards.

Abduction A movement away from the mid-line of the body, such as when the arm is lifted sideways away from the body.

Adduction A movement towards the mid-line of the body, such as when the arm is returned closer to the body after being abducted.

Circumduction A movement in a circular direction, for example, arm circling is circumduction at the shoulder joint.

Proximal Moving a body part closer to the trunk, or nearer to the point of origin of the body part.

Distal Moving a body part away from the trunk, or from the point of origin of a body part.

ANATOMICAL POSITIONS

Superior Towards the head, or upper, or above.

Inferior Towards the feet, or lower, or below.

Anterior Front, or in front of.

Posterior Back, or at the back of.

Medial Towards the mid-line of the body.

Lateral Towards, or on the outside of the body.

Supine Lying face upwards.

Prone Lying face downwards.

2 — MUSCLE FITNESS

Not taking care of our muscles on a daily basis can lead to many health problems. Being overweight, obesity, heart complaints or high blood pressure, in addition to poor self-esteem and bouts of lethargy in our daily activities, are but a few reasons to keep fit. What shape we are in, both physically and mentally, is directly influenced by how we take care of our muscles on a daily basis and on our general level of fitness. In this chapter the three principles of muscle fitness: exercise, stretching and nutrition are also outlined.

DAILY MUSCLE CARE

There are three essentials for developing and maintaining muscle health:

1. *Regular exercise* which helps us maintain a basic level of fitness. Being physically fit promotes heart and lung (cardiovascular) fitness as well as developing basic muscle strength.
2. *Stretching* which practised on a regular basis helps retain flexibility in your muscles and helps avoid them tightening.
3. *Nutrition* which is vital for all living tissue and muscles are no exception. A healthy lifestyle and balanced diet are vital for muscle health.

Let us review these three important aspects of muscle fitness in more detail.

Regular exercise

'Physical fitness' is defined as having enough energy to perform your daily duties with energy left at the end of each day to enjoy your leisure time.

While this is a very general definition, it accurately depicts a non-scientific way of assessing our individual fitness. Have you ever noticed that on days when you do not exercise at all, such as when sitting at a desk all day, that you are more lethargic than the times you have been physically active all day? This is why it is critical to get into the habit of regularly exercising, because once you stop, it is much harder to return to a regular fitness programme.

On a more scientific level, measuring your heart rate via your pulse can be a helpful measure of your fitness. As you gain fitness your resting heart rate

24

should decrease. The ideal time to take your heart rate is first thing in the morning. It can be taken by placing the third and fourth fingers on the side of the neck. Here you can easily detect the carotid artery pulse.

The average heart rate for a sedentary man is around 72 bpm (beats per minute), and for a woman it is around 80 bpm. These rates are significantly lower in the trained athlete and may go as low as 30–40 bpm.

If you wanted to find out even more about your level of fitness, you could get a complete fitness evaluation from a qualified fitness instructor or exercise scientist. These people are often employed by gymnasiums, sports science or sports medicine clinics. The evaluation may involve a stress, or sub-maximal test using a bicycle or treadmill as an ergonometer (the machine you are tested on). However, these tests are usually more suitable for the élite athlete as they test the exercising muscle's ability to use oxygen and determine how intensively you can push your body. Tests provided by gyms such as the Harvard step test or PWC 170 are sufficient for most individuals.

What you need to decide is what you really want to know about yourself. If you just wish to know your areas of weakness (such as the areas which are inflexible and so on), getting yourself a postural assessment may be sufficient. However, if you would like to monitor how you are progressing over a period of time with your fitness programme, the aforementioned tests, provided by many gymnasiums, would be ideal.

Aerobic and anaerobic exercise

The most effective form of exercise for long term cardiovascular fitness is called aerobic exercise. This means breathing in air and oxygen continuously to supply the working muscle. Examples of aerobic exercise are jogging, walking and swimming.

Other exercise, called anaerobic exercise, does not utilise oxygen, but uses energy stores from within the muscle, for instance, glycogen. Sprinting is an example of anaerobic exercise. Have you noticed how a sprinter breathes heavily at the end of a race? A jogger rarely does this at the end of a run, as oxygen is available throughout the jog because of its lower level of intensity.

While both forms of exercise are excellent for fitness, aerobic exercise is essential for improving physical fitness in the long term. The heart and lungs are stressed continuously over a longer period of time so these organs improve in their efficiency. The efficiency of the heart and lungs thus determines our general level of fitness. Anaerobic exercise, alternatively, is usually performed in short bursts and contributes more to specific fitness for each sport. To be able to perform well during anaerobic activity, however, you have to improve your basic level of aerobic fitness. For instance, if you play tennis socially but decide to combine this with a regular aerobic walking programme, you will not be so tired after your social tennis games as you will be aerobically fitter, and therefore able to cope with the anaerobic exercise much more easily.

Starting a fitness programme

If you are not used to exercising regularly, the following guidelines will help you to decide what activity is appropriate for you, and for how long and how often you should do it.

Firstly, if you are over 30 and have not exercised for some years, it would be advisable to see your doctor for a medical check-up to screen for any medical precautions you may need to take. This is particularly important if you are older, heavier, lead a sedentary lifestyle or are a male with a type A personality (highly stressed, and driven in your work, personal or sporting life). The traits of a type A male are high risk factors which can lead to health problems such as heart complaints or high blood pressure.

Aside from this there are a few basic hints to follow when you are trying to get fit. Using the letters FITT we can outline the main things you need to consider when taking up an aerobic exercise programme.

Frequency To gain cardiovascular fitness you need to exercise a minimum of three to four times each week. It is best to try to exercise every second day as opposed to exercising for a few days and then doing no exercise for the rest of the week.

Intensity You need to exercise at 60–80 per cent of your maximum heart rate (MHR) to achieve a cardiovascular training effect. Your MHR can be estimated by subtracting your age from 220. The fitter you are, the higher the percentage of your MHR it is safe to work at.

For instance, if you are 40 years old and very unfit then you need to work at approximately 60 per cent of your MHR. This would be between 105 and 110 bpm (0.60 × 180). However, if you are working at greater than 80–85 per cent of your MHR, you are more likely to be working anaerobically. This is because there is not enough time for the oxygen breathed in to pass from the lungs to the exercising muscle, and the muscle must therefore utilise energy stores from within the muscle. It is difficult to sustain this level of exercise for extended periods of time. This differs from aerobic exercise, where there is adequate time by the exercising muscle to utilise the oxygen taken in with each breath. To achieve a general level of cardiovascular fitness, aerobic exercise, performed at 60–80 per cent of your MHR is advised. To supplement your training, anaerobic exercises (80–85 per cent MHR) are recommended.

However, it is the lower level, sustained exercise that achieves weight loss if this is your goal, not the high intensity, high-speed workouts performed in short bursts. This latter form of workout, though, is important to include if your particular sport or activity requires anaerobic work such as squash or football. If you are uncertain what level you are exercising at, take your carotid artery pulse for 10 seconds. Trying to maintain contact for the entire 60 seconds is often difficult if you are exercising. Once you have a figure, then multiply this by six. This will give you an idea of what range of the 60–85 per cent of your MHR you are working in.

The 'whistle' test is another helpful way of assessing if you are working out at too intense a level. This involves whistling or talking while you jog or walk. If you are unable to, then you are probably working at too high a heart rate and may be working anaerobically.

Basically, aerobic exercise is the ideal for heart/lung fitness but combined with anaerobic exercise, will provide an even more balanced programme.

Type To gain long term cardiovascular fitness, as stated previously, you need to choose an exercise that works you aerobically. Examples of aerobic exercise are jogging, brisk walking, cycling, swimming and some fitness, dance or aquarobics classes. Using weights in circuit training classes is also aerobic. Anaerobic activities include sprinting, tennis and squash. There can, however, be variations in these categorisations. Very fit squash players may work aerobically throughout most of their game but have bursts of anaerobic work during the match. The key to working effectively aerobically is that the workout must be continuous — that is, if you are doing lap swimming you must minimise the breaks you have between laps and try to aim for consistency in your workout.

The key to your choice of exercise, though, is that you must enjoy it. Try to vary your fitness routine. Variation in your fitness programme is a must for staying motivated if you are just beginning it. For example, combining swimming, jogging and tennis may suit some. Others, however, may prefer the routine involved in doing just one particular activity. You must also choose what you can fit into your daily lifestyle. Be realistic about the type of exercise you choose. Starting a swimming programme in the middle of winter is not a good incentive for staying motivated!

Time To be effective in your workout you need to maintain your elevated heart rate for a minimum of 15–20 minutes. In anaerobic activities it is difficult to sustain this level continuously for this length of time. Ideally your workout should be about half an hour so you can include a warm-up and cool-down in your exercise routine.

Stretching

Stretching refers to the elongation that occurs when the origin and insertion of a muscle are moved as far away as possible from each other. Stretching improves the flexibility of the muscle and the underlying joint.

Strengthening, alternatively, refers to when the muscle is repeatedly contracted against resistance, either through range or within a fixed range. This may cause hypertrophy, or enlargement of the muscle belly. Strengthening may be achieved by working the body against gravity, for instance, raising the head and shoulders off the floor to strengthen the abdominals when doing a bent-leg sit-up, or by using specific weights.

While the mechanisms of strengthening are quite well understood, clinical findings by health professionals and personal reasons by the individual for stretching, far outweigh any scientific reasons for stretching. In fact, the latter barely exist. Then why stretch? Stretching is advocated as a means to increase flexibility; improve blood supply to the muscle; for relaxation; to improve biomechanical efficiency; to improve co-ordination between muscle groups; to decrease muscle tightening after physical activity, particularly in sports such as weight training; to improve posture; and last but not least, to prevent injury and decrease the muscle tightening effect that occurs with age.

Improving flexibility means joints may be moved through a greater range. This can enhance sporting performance. By practising the stretches shown in this book, your improvement in muscle tone and general flexibility should soon become self-evident. Stretching should at all times be balanced by a strengthening programme to ensure you do not overstretch already lengthened muscles. Poor posture may lead to tightening and overlengthening of muscles. Chapter 3 will clarify how this effect may be counteracted and corrected.

When to stretch

Stretching should be performed daily as well as being incorporated in both the warm-up and cool-down phase of your sport or activity. Stretching after a loosening of the muscles by gentle exercise is ideal. That is, try not to stretch when you are cold and have not loosened up at all.

The stretch reflex

When a muscle is suddenly stretched, a reflex comes into play which causes the muscle to involuntarily contract. This is known as the stretch reflex. If you were to suddenly stretch again, while the muscle was contracted, this would damage the myofibrils of the muscle, causing microtears, resulting in fibrous or scar tissue. This is why bouncing while touching your toes is considered harmful to the muscles of the lower back — aside from the load placed on the discs of the lumbar region of the spine.

How to stretch

There are basically five types of stretching. These are:

1. **Static stretching** which takes the muscle to the end of its range and when this position is held for the minimum 6–10 seconds, the stretch reflex is actually inhibited. Therefore, the muscle relaxes and permits more range and an increased muscle length. This should be repeated about three times, each time moving gently into a new range. Breathing out as you are stretching the muscles, assists the body to relax and improves the effectiveness of your stretching. The longer a stretch is held, the more effective the increase in muscle length.

2. **Dynamic stretching** is a type of stretching which refers to faster movements where the muscle is gradually worked to its full range. This type of stretching is used a lot in the martial arts. An example where dynamic stretching is applicable is for a full-back in rugby union. It would be inappropriate for this player to simply do static stretching of the hamstrings prior to play. To prepare the leg muscles for the high kicks required in this position of play, the hamstrings must be gradually taken to their full range. This is done by dynamically stretching them at an increasing speed, but *not bouncing* the movement at the end of

range. This could be achieved by bringing the bent knee up to the chest, while standing, and progressing this gradually to straight leg, high kicks.

3. **Ballistic stretching** This refers to fast, jerky movements, where a double bounce is performed at the end of range of a movement, such as bouncing when touching your toes. This type of stretching is not recommended for most sports because of the potential tearing of myofibrils it may cause which, in the long term, only serves to reduce the effectiveness of your stretching because of the scar tissue created. However, performed in a controlled manner, just short of the end-range of a movement, dancers and gymnasts may incorporate some ballistic stretching to prepare them for their action. For all other sports, ballistic stretching is *not* recommended.

4. **PNF (Proprioceptive neuromuscular facilitation) stretching** This type of stretching has been shown to be the most effective way to increase muscle length. It involves doing a static stretch, followed by an isometric contraction (see page 69) of the muscle against an immovable resistance — your own hands or a partner's — for 6–10 seconds. Then the muscle is relaxed and gently taken into its new range. It is best to repeat this about three times.

The following precautions should be observed with PNF stretching:

- It should only be attempted after a total body warm-up.
- The isometric contraction should never be explosive, that is, started suddenly. The resistance should be slowly increased.
- A partner should only provide resistance in the isometric phase, and only guide and not force the muscle in the static stretch phase.
- The isometric contraction should involve a gradual increase in effort in the first 2 seconds which is then sustained for an additional 4–6 seconds.

5. **Range of movement stretching** This type of stretching simply refers to taking a muscle through the full range which the underlying joint permits. (It can be done in aquarobics classes.) It is also part of the overall concept included in Tai Chi and in Feldenkrais exercise movements (see Suggested Reading List). Working with a practitioner skilled in these forms of health disciplines is ideal to learn these movement patterns.

Proprioceptive neuromuscular facilitation (PNF) and range of movement stretching are considered to be the most effective. Fast, jerky ballistic stretching is not recommended as this can cause damage to the muscle because of the stretch reflex.

Try the different methods to find which form of stretching works best for you. Try to work with a partner whenever possible.

Hypermobility — overflexibility

Have you noticed how some people are able to touch their toes; even put their hands or elbows on the floor while you are struggling to touch your knees? While it may seem wonderful that someone can be so flexible, it does have its disadvantages.

When someone is more flexible than normal it is called being *hypermobile*.

(Some people mistakenly call this being double jointed, which is anatomically incorrect.) With hypermobility, due to increased muscle length and ligament laxity, the joints can move far further than they normally can. Some people are hypermobile throughout all their joints while others have specific joint hypermobility. The latter usually occurs at the wrist, being able to bend the fingers back onto the forearm, or of the thumb, where it too is able to be brought back up to the forearm.

Other joints where this may occur are the elbows and knees. Both are able to extend (called hyperextension) past 180 degrees. This is considered to be the normal range at the hinge joints of the knees and the elbow.

Specific joint hypermobility should pose no problems. However, sometimes at the knees it can. If, when you stand, your knees tend to curve backwards and lock back, try to bend them slightly, otherwise postural problems in the spine can develop as the upper back attempts to compensate for this excessive mobility in the lower limb.

General hypermobility should not be a problem. However, while this type of flexibility is almost a prerequisite for gymnasts or dancers, if you do not exercise regularly, but have inherent, general hypermobility, instability around joints can develop. When young, this may not be a problem, but with age, if strength in the muscles is not retained, or if excess weight is carried, stress on joints can be far greater than it is for the inflexible person. An analogy would be trying to drive the car but loosening all the bolts that keep the tyres secure. Just as this would be risky, so is our body vulnerable when excessive joint mobility, usually due to ligament laxity, is not balanced by adequate strength.

The reasons for hypermobility are not fully understood. Genetics appears sometimes to play a role, but the type of sport or physical activities we are exposed to as children appears to be more influential. For instance, if you did gymnastics or ballet in your adolescent years, your chances of being flexible are greater than if you did no stretching or flexibility work.

Probably the biggest problem for people who are hypermobile is if they return to sport after a few years' break of no regular fitness activity. Fitness instructors who take aerobics classes are often classic examples of this. When they start to take classes after a long break, the high impact and jumping soon stresses their unstable joints which no longer have the strength, balance and control around them as they used to. Clunking joints, particularly hips, may be indicative of instability in a joint (or of muscle imbalance) and this often occurs in hypermobile people. The good news is that hypermobility need not be a problem, but certainly retaining strength of all muscles is critical to maintaining stability around your joints, if you are hypermobile.

Nutrition

There are so many facts and fallacies in the area of nutrition. Do you know anybody who is interested in health and fitness who does not take an active interest in the latest diet, the latest mineral or vitamin supplement and so on? While it is a very important aspect of muscle fitness it should not become an obsession. This only leads to negative side effects in the body.

The key to healthy eating is not getting attached to some particular fad, but eating lighter, nutritious meals on a regular basis. If weight loss is your goal, remember if too few kilojoules are consumed your body readjusts to this by slowing down its basal metabolic rate (BMR). This is the basic amount of energy required by the body to keep it functioning. Therefore, as soon as you start to eat normally, you will only put on any weight that you have lost because the body will use the kilojoules you take in at a much slower rate. Furthermore, short term weight loss is usually just fluid loss and not fatty tissue!

Basically, if one is overweight, then this simply means too many kilojoules are being taken in compared with the number that are being used up. The excess is stored as fat. It is important, therefore, to consider the type of food one is eating. One can still eat a healthy and hearty sized meal without eating extra kilojoules. Learning the type of foods high in kilojoules can assist in the planning of meals. Unfortunately, it is usually the highly refined sweets, loaded in kilojoules, that we often eat in between meals, which give us our short term energy boosters.

For the most part though, being overweight does not come from overeating per se but from the poor dietary habits one develops to cope with emotional or mental stress, or simply boredom. Exercising regularly, being content in one's job and practising relaxation techniques whenever possible, all assist in improving one's self-esteem — which in turn means one will not wish to overeat.

Changing dietary habits will not happen in a day, but understanding how to change them is a starting point. *The Muscle Fitness Book* will not even attempt to cover this controversial and broad spectrumed issue. Refer to the Suggested Reading List to find out some places where common sense information can be found on dealing with food daily from both a physical and mental viewpoint.

COMMONLY ASKED QUESTIONS

What happens to muscles with age?

Skeletal muscles are either postural or phasic depending on their function. With age, postural muscles — those that support us in standing, sitting and lying — tend to tighten, while phasic muscles — that is those that are more active when we are in motion — tend to weaken. Examples of postural muscles are: the calves, hamstrings, back extensors and iliopsoas (a hip flexor) and the pectorals in the upper limb. Examples of phasic muscles are: the quadriceps, abdominals and tibialis anterior. However, depending on how we stand, and our postural type (see page 40) — this determines how muscles are used. That is, muscles that should be postural may not be being used properly and therefore may not have the tone they should have.

However, unfortunately all muscles do tend to lose tone as we age. The supportive connective tissue and fascia which surrounds, interconnects and supports muscles and other structures also loses its elasticity. Usually beyond the age of 30 this process becomes more prevalent. Maintaining good posture can retain healthy tone in our muscles and not permit the process of our bodies giving into gravity, resulting in the sagging look our muscles can sometimes have as we become older. Also, with age, muscles that are not used regularly not only tend to lose tone but also tend to accumulate fat. The abdomen and thighs are classic examples of this. It must be noted though that fat deposition is obviously influenced by other factors such as diet and hormones. For instance, for child-bearing reasons women are thought to gain fat on the thighs and buttocks, while men for unknown reasons tend to gain fat on the stomach.

In summary, it does seem the key to preventing our muscles from ageing is a combination of regular exercise, stretching and sound nutrition.

Are muscles of females and males the same?

While the basic physiological properties of muscle are the same for both sexes, more general aspects regarding body composition differ, creating the visible differences between males and females. The three significant body differences to note are: strength and size, fat and flexibility.

Strength

Because of the male hormone testosterone, males do tend to bulk — that is, increase the size of their muscles more readily — particularly when they engage in a weight training programme. However, research by Wilmore (see Suggested Reading List) indicates that when women undertake weight training there is minimal difference in strength when this is measured in proportion to body weight. However, without strength-training, women's strength is generally found to be 25–28 per cent lower than men's. Women used to worry that they might bulk if they used weights. However, unless women have a higher than normal level of testosterone they will increase strength and improve tone with weight training but not significantly bulk. The taking of steroids will obviously create undesirable bulking — for both sexes.

Fat differences

Women have a generally higher content of fat in their bodies. The average fat content for a young, healthy, adult male is 10–15 per cent, and for a young, healthy, adult woman it is 16–25 per cent. As we age, men and women have 5–10 per cent more fat than their younger counterparts. However the increase in body fat with age is not solely physiological but is also lifestyle related.

Physical activity and level of fitness directly influence body fat content. According to Wilmore variations of between 4–20 per cent for male athletes and 10–26 per cent for female athletes may exist. The type of sporting activity and the amount of physical training involved are the main determinants of body composition in élite athletes.

Approximate levels of fat content can be gained by the use of fat calipers, used by specialists who do fitness testing. A more accurate figure can be determined by underwater weighing used at sports science research laboratories.

Flexibility

As a rule, women tend to be more flexible than men. While female hormones are claimed to contribute to this, and bearing in mind we all have our own skeletal and anatomical limitations, males can improve their flexibility. However, in the later years it is certainly more difficult to improve flexibility than when younger — for males particularly more so than women. Physiological changes in connective tissue contribute markedly to the stiffness that occurs with age — more so than sex-related reasons. In other words, the more we exercise and stretch, the more chance we have of reducing the predisposition we have to becoming stiff and tight in our joints and less flexible as we age (both males and females).

The main difference in flexibility between the sexes is most obvious during pregnancy. Due to the presence of the hormone relaxin in the female body, ligaments become more lax, predominantly in the pelvic region, the hips and the lower back. This is why it is important to maintain strength throughout pregnancy — swimming is ideal. Likewise after birth, ligaments take a few months to regain their normal physiological properties so post-natal fitness is critical as soon as is medically recommended.

Are children's and adults' muscles the same?

The basic molecular and physiological structure of adults' and children's muscles is the same. What differs is obviously the ability of children's muscle to grow and lengthen as the underlying growth plates in the bones alter, permitting growth in height. One marked difference between adults' and children's musculoskeletal systems is the relative elasticity of children's tissues. Ligaments, which support joints, do not reach maturity till late adolescence. This means children tend to be more flexible than adults — or at least, should be! Similarly, the connective tissue (the non-contractile part of a muscle) is less fibrous and has more fluid when we are younger. Damage to any of these soft tissues also repairs more quickly. It is not normal for a child to be stiff and inflexible. However, being introduced to excessive flexibility work as a child can also cause problems in later life. (See page 156.)

Are growing pains in children real?

Controversy still surrounds the answer to this question. A suggested reason for growing pains is an imbalance in the rate of growth of the bone compared with the rate of muscle growth.

This certainly seems possible when we consider that most children get these pains during growth-spurt phases — that is, when they are growing at a rate much quicker than normal. Basically though, pain is the body's way of telling us something is wrong, so do not ignore the child's complaints. Often children may complain of pain in their joints. If it is knee pain it may be because they are doing too much jumping or running for their age and the quadriceps tendon (the muscle down the front of the thigh) is pulling on the growth plate of the tibia (shin bone). A large lump may begin to appear. If this occurs, seek advice and treatment from a sports specialist. It must be attended to as early as possible to prevent musculoskeletal problems in later life.

Children who complain of lower back, hip or feet pain may have a skeletal problem such as leg length difference, flat feet, or a muscle imbalance where a scoliosis or a lordosis (often incorrectly called a sway back) may develop. A postural assessment from a physiotherapist at this age, and recommended exercises will lessen the predisposition children may have to getting problems later.

Referral to a podiatrist (a specialist who deals with feet problems) may be necessary if you notice your children developing strange habits when they are walking, or if they excessively wear down one particular part of their shoes. Corns and bunions in children's (and of course, adults') feet are a certain sign of imbalance further up the body — usually the knees, hip or spine.

Whatever the reason though, growing pains *are* usually real. If the ache is specific to particular muscle groups, particularly of the weight-bearing joints, muscle tightness, weakness or imbalance may be present. A postural assessment will screen for this. Weight-bearing, that is standing, sitting, running and so on, actually stimulates the growth of bone. Therefore, it is unusual to get growing pains in the upper limb. The exception is in teenage girls who may suffer thoracic or mid-upper back pains as their bust is developing. Poor posture which often results at this age is very difficult to correct later on, so this is the time to subtly assist the teenager to become aware of the principles of good posture.

Consult a doctor if a child complains of generalised aches all through the body. It may not be a problem of musculoskeletal origin.

A final point with children is that genetics do play a part in determining body type, to an extent. Features such as being tall and thin, short and plump, bow-legged and so on, are not easy to alter. (See Figure 2.1.) However intervention in the teenage years can minimise the tendency for children to adopt their parents' skeletal characteristics, such as stooping forward or slumped posture. Rather than genetic influence it would seem children tend to adopt patterns and simulate how their parents move and stand. Therefore, it is probably ineffective to try and alter a child's posture if the parent's stance is not good! Reminding a child to stand up straight if the parent's posture is poor is probably no use.

Why do some people seem to have strong muscles while others cannot seem to build their muscles up no matter how much they weight train or exercise?

Unfortunately for most of us, some people do tend to be more naturally muscle bound than others. The scientific term for how a muscle appears and feels is called its muscle tone. Two major factors influencing both muscle size and overall muscle shape are body type and muscle tone. Both of these are clarified below.

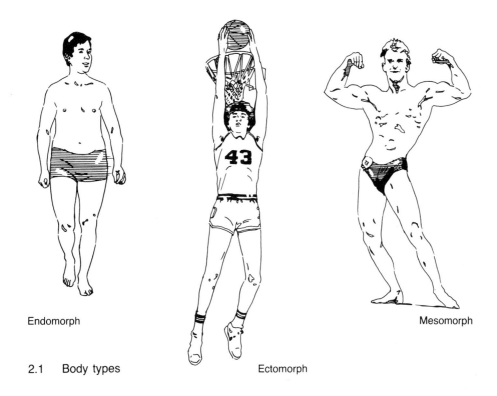

Endomorph

Mesomorph

2.1   Body types   Ectomorph

Body type

Body shape may be classified into three groups: *ectomorph* (tall and thin), *meso-morph* (muscular), and *endomorph* (a tendency to be short and plump). (See Figure 2.1.)

Most of us have attributes from each body type but basically it is more difficult for a tall, thin person to build up muscle bulk just as it is difficult to expect an endomorph to try and achieve unnatural slimness. Accepting realistically what our body type is will assist us in determining our long term goals with respect to exercise and sport. For instance, short, plump people do not make good basketballers as tall, thin people do not make good hookers in rugby. Fortunately, as a rule we tend to choose sports suitable for our body types.

Muscle tone

Not only does body type determine muscle tone but how we use our muscles can determine the tone, or 'tautness' or 'firmness' of a muscle. A tall, thin person who stands poorly may look like he or she has a protruding stomach, flat, toneless hamstrings and calves, and a poked forward chin. Corrective postural measures and appropriate exercise can restore good tone to all these muscles by simply using them correctly again! Chapter 3 deals solely with postural analysis and the concept of muscle balance.

3 — MUSCLES AND POSTURE

To achieve muscle fitness, a balance of strength and flexibility between muscle groups is essential. In our daily lifestyle muscles are often not used through their full range. This leads to an increase in connective tissue (the non-contractile component of the muscle) within the muscle belly, and causes resultant shortening and tightening. If this imbalance becomes chronic, poor posture can develop in the long term because of the abnormal load placed on underlying joints. Muscles are said to be in a state of 'dysfunction' when they are not working through their fully effective range. This in turn significantly impedes the efficiency with which we carry out, not only activities of daily living, but even more importantly, can markedly limit our sporting performance.

This chapter will review what is meant by ideal posture and good muscle balance. Six typical postural types are outlined and the key to correction shown. You should be able to design your own daily exercise programme from this classification. Chapter 7 provides exercises for postural correction. These exercises, when performed daily, will help you to improve your posture as well as ultimately provide you with a more efficient body for playing and enjoying your sport.

Some of the terms used when discussing posture are clarified below.

ANATOMICAL TERMS

Cervical The upper seven vertebrae in the neck.

Thoracic The twelve vertebrae which attach to the ribs.

Lumbar The lower five vertebrae.

Lumbosacral The junction where the lumbar vertebrae meet the sacrum. The lowest five vertebrae which are fused together comprise this bone.

Greater trochanter The bony prominence on the outside of the thigh (the femur).

Patella The knee-cap.

Lateral malleolus The bony prominence on the outside of the ankle.

POSTURAL TERMINOLOGY

Kyphosis An outward curve of the spine which usually occurs in the thoracic spine.

Lordosis An excessive inward curve in the spine, which usually occurs at the lumbar or cervical region.

Scoliosis An s-shape bend which can be seen when viewing the spine posteriorly.

Handedness pattern Refers to being right- or left-handed and the subsequent postural pattern that develops.

IDEAL POSTURE

Posture refers to how we hold our bodies. The type of work we do, sporting activities, personality, emotions, heredity, disease and our height are all major influences on our posture.

Ideal posture occurs when all body parts are balanced and in alignment with each other. Ida Rolf (see Suggested Reading List) developed a static model of body parts where she compared the segments of the body (head, thorax, pelvis and legs) with a pile of blocks. (See Figure 3.1.) When these blocks are piled securely over each other, the structure is stable. The weight of each part is carried evenly by the parts below. The ball and socket joint of the hips permits us to carry the heavier weight of the upper torso on the relatively smaller base provided by our feet.

Muscles should work minimally if alignment is good. However, due to our sedentary lifestyle and other extrinsic factors such as high-heels, poor nutrition or lack of fitness, muscle tightness and weakness can develop, creating an abnormal load and stress on underlying parts. Most of us spend a lifetime with a body that is imbalanced. The high incidence of back pain in our community clearly reflects this. Another excellent analogy to describe ideal posture is to compare the body with a radio tower. The steel structure is analogous to the bones, and the muscles and their associated connective tissue are the guy wires. Both are important for the stability of the tower or the body.

Poor posture, or imbalance in the body, creates much the same effect on the body as on a tent with uneven pull on all its ropes. In much the same way, muscles influence our posture.

MUSCLE BALANCE

Basically then, our body can be compared to any machine. While movement is balanced, efficient and free-flowing, problems are minimal. Imbalance, however, can lead to creaky, clunky or clicky joints and ultimately, pain. Therefore, how muscles establish balance around our joints is of prime importance. A balanced programme of stretching and strengthening provides the fine tuning our body requires. Each joint in the body must have complete freedom in all the directions which the joint permits, or stiffness will develop.

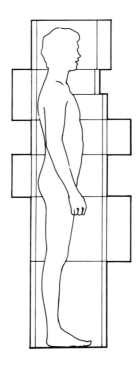

3.1   Rolf's block model

When one block is pushed forward, for instance, the head and neck, another must be pushed back or twisted at another level to compensate.

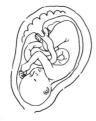

**Posture in the womb
(c-shaped curve)**

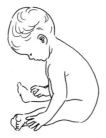

Sitting posture before neck curve develops

3.2   Development of the curves of the spine

For example, the shoulder is a ball and socket joint, but if we tighten up one side of this joint by overdeveloping and shortening our pectoralis major and pectoralis minor, imbalance around the joint creating a rounded shoulder look will result. Weakness of the abdominals (the stomach muscles), excessive push-ups, bench press work or bent-leg sit-ups, can also cause this effect. Imbalance such as this can place stress on surrounding and underlying structures such as the neck or the thoracic spine.

Ideal posture is when there is a balance in the body between all muscle groups. When standing, a plumb line should fall through the middle of the ear, middle of the shoulder, middle of the femur and down to slightly behind the lateral malleolus. (See Figure 3.5.)

MUSCLE IMBALANCE

Muscle imbalance readily develops around our joints and places undue load on underlying structures, when the inevitable process of tightening and weakening is hastened by sedentary lifestyle or by imbalanced exercise programmes. Regular exercise and positive self-awareness can minimise our predisposition to muscle imbalance.

Spinal curvature

Curves in our spine are normal; excessive curves are not. One fallacy is that the curves in our spine predispose us to neck and back pain. This is not the case as the curves in our spine are essential to enable us to maintain an upright stance. Excessive curves may predispose us to problems, however. How the body develops its curves illustrates how necessary they are for the maintenance of an upright stance and bipedal gait.

When we are born the spine has a c-shaped curve, such as it had when the foetus was developing in the womb. (See Figure 3.1.)

After several months, as the child tries sitting, he or she learns to lift the relatively heavy head back into an upright position, to be able to see ahead. While balance is still poor, the legs are spread wide to provide a wide triangular base for support. (See Figure 3.2.)

As the child tries to stand he or she uses objects to assist in stability. A curve in the lower back (called the lumbar curve) gradually develops to bring the head over the centre of gravity. As the child's balance improves these curves become less marked.

However, because of our sedentary lifestyle and misuse of muscles, the load borne through these curves is often unnecessarily increased. Abnormal stress is placed on joints and this can result in pain.

People's height can significantly influence the curves in the spine and the type of posture the individual develops. Unfortunately, everything in our environment is designed for the 'average' height person. Subsequently, the tall and short have to make postural adjustments to fit into their surroundings — be it at home, the office, the car, or wherever.

As a result, people who are short spend most of their lives looking upwards and often develop an excessive curve in their cervical or lumbar region. (See Figure 3.3.) An excessive inward curve is called a *lordosis*.

Tall, or above normal height people, tend to find everything is too low for them and are always having to look downwards. Tall people tend to develop an extra outward curve usually in the thoracic spine. This is called a *kyphosis*. (See Figure 3.4.)

When there is an excessive s-shape in the spine (when we are assessing it from behind) this is called a *scoliosis*. This may be postural, that is due to muscle imbalance, or structural, resulting, for instance, from leg length difference.

POSTURAL TYPES

Most people, whether short or tall, can be classified into one of the following categories defined by Kendall and McCreary (the pioneers of postural analysis in the 1950s).

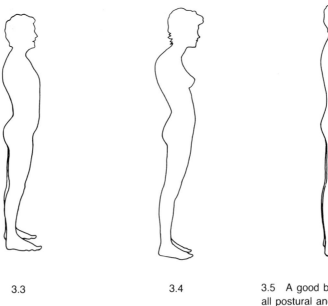

3.3   3.4   3.5 A good balance between
all postural and phasic muscles.
Plumb line should ideally drop
through the middle of the ear,
3.3   Posture frequently developed by the short   the shoulder, the hips, the knees
3.4   Posture frequently developed by the tall   and finish slightly anterior to
3.5   Ideal posture   the lateral malleolus.

Try to identify which classification you feel you may be. You may have components of a few of the types, but nonetheless, you should be able to find the key to correcting your posture and establish the exercises that are the most suitable for you.

The six postural types are:

1. Ideal
2. Lordosis
3. Kyphosis/lordosis
4. Flat back
5. Sway back
6. Military

The most common types of postures seen today are the kyphosis or kyphosis/lordosis and the sway back. Each of these is shown on the following pages and the major features creating the imbalance are noted. (Chapter 7 provides all the exercises for postural correction.) The key to the exercises is to alter one's awareness of how the body is routinely used in poor habitual patterns. It is not how many of the exercises you do that matters, but how well you do them. While you may not change your body type by doing the specified exercises, you can minimise the stress being placed on your joints by your poor posture. Once you have chosen the most suitable exercises for yourself be sure to combine these with the exercises and stretches appropriate to your particular sport. Consult a sports specialist who does postural assessment if you are uncertain what type of posture you have. Postural balance is critical to achieve the optimum performance from your body when you are playing a sport.

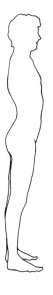

Pelvis anteriorly tilted

Weak lower abdominals
and external obliques

Tight back muscles (extensors)
Tight hip flexors, iliopsoas, quadriceps and hip abductors

Tight and weak hamstrings

3.6   Lordosis

Ideal

Key feature: Balance, poise and symmetry. Dancers often achieve ideal posture.

Lordosis

Key feature: An inwardly curved or lordosed lower back.

Key to correction:

- To strengthen abdominals, particularly the lower abdominals. By strengthening the external oblique, the pelvis is able to be maintained in a more posteriorly tilted position.
- All posterior musculature requires stretching. Particularly the lower back, the hamstrings and usually the calves. Hip flexors including iliopsoas, rectus fermoris and hip abductors (tensor fascia latae) usually need stretching.

Specific awareness exercise: Try to always think tall, while softening and relaxing your knees. That is, do not stand with your knees locked back. It may be helpful to imagine your rib cage is lifting up and away from your lower stomach while gently tilting your pelvis backwards. Your stomach muscles should not need to be held taut to flatten your back. They should be strong enough to do this and still be relaxed.

On a daily basis, if you have a lordotic posture, avoid doing exercises which encourage excessive hyperextension of the back, either passive or active, and do not use a back support or chair where you rest on your knees and shins which encourages this inward curve of the back. Let the inward curve of the lower back flex a little (do not slump though), and relax when you sit.

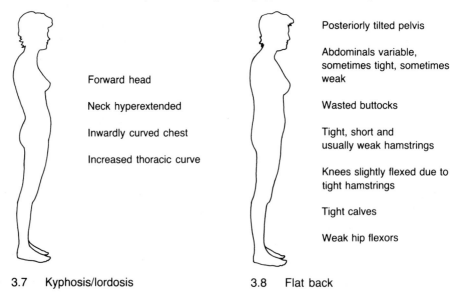

Forward head

Neck hyperextended

Inwardly curved chest

Increased thoracic curve

Posteriorly tilted pelvis

Abdominals variable, sometimes tight, sometimes weak

Wasted buttocks

Tight, short and usually weak hamstrings

Knees slightly flexed due to tight hamstrings

Tight calves

Weak hip flexors

3.7   Kyphosis/lordosis   3.8   Flat back

Kyphosis / lordosis

Key features: An outwardly curved, convex thoracic spine and an inwardly curved lower back. Often an inwardly curved cervical spine develops to compensate. This is a common postural type adopted by the sedentary desk worker or by tall people.

Key to correction:

For kyphosis: Need to improve mobility of the shoulders and thoracic spine. Increase thoracic spine extension, stretch the thoracic spine and strengthen the thoracic spine while standing.

For cervical lordosis: being aware of tucking the chin in and lengthening the back of the neck can reduce this poked forward position of the neck.

For kyphosis/lordosis: For this postural type the aim is to increase mid- and upper back extension, while increasing lower back flexion. Lower abdominal strengthening and external oblique strengthening to reduce excessive lumbar lordosis is essential. All shoulder flexibility work needs to be done while maintaining a posteriorly tilted pelvis.

Specific exercise: Try to hold a piece of paper under the chin, flatten the back of your neck and think of these upper neck muscles being stretched tall. Be sure to relax once you have done this. Do not let tension in your muscles remain once you have corrected your posture, that is, you should not be trying too hard, otherwise you will fatigue your muscles and you will return to your old posture.

Another ideal exercise is to stand with your back against a wall, flatten the lumbar spine and stretch the arms above the head, until they can reach the wall with the back still flattened. This is a good exercise to assess how your posture is improving. This should be done as many times a day as possible.

Avoid prolonged sitting, take breaks where possible if you have a sedentary occupation and do the above-mentioned wall exercise for stretching and strengthening the shoulders and upper back musculature whenever possible.

Flatback

Key feature: No lumbar curve. Usually a kyphosis of the upper thoracic spine exists.

Key to correction:

- To try and develop a normal lumbar or lower back curve and maintain this while standing, sitting and in all daily activities.
- Hamstrings need stretching while maintaining a lordosed lumbar curve. This can be achieved by straightening the leg when sitting.
- Back muscles may be strong, but gluteus maximus may need strengthening.

Specific exercise: when sitting, practise shifting the weight off the buttocks

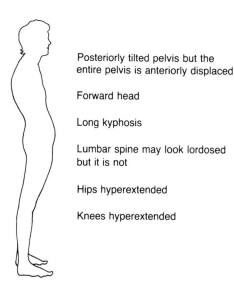

Posteriorly tilted pelvis but the
entire pelvis is anteriorly displaced

Forward head

Long kyphosis

Lumbar spine may look lordosed
but it is not

Hips hyperextended

Knees hyperextended

Shoulders pulled up and back

Tight lordosed thoraco-lumbar
spine

Both postural and phasic
muscles appear taut and tight

Tight and shortened hamstrings
and calves

Often tight hip flexors

3.9   Sway back   3.10   Military

and shifting the upper body forward by trying to tilt the lower back inwards, creating a lordosis. Using a lumbar roll (a back support which can be bought from chemists) when sitting will help you increase your lumbar curve. Using a chair where your weight is taken through your shins and knees will encourage the development of a normal lumbar curve.

Sway back

Key feature: this posture looks deceptively like the lordosed posture but differs in that the entire pelvis and top end of the thighs are swayed forward in relation to the feet. To counteract the position of the pelvis the upper body is swayed back. Hence the term 'sway back' is used for this postural type. Hypermobile people — those who are over flexible — tend to adopt this posture if they do not have adequate strength in their muscles to support their joints. They basically rely on the ligaments of their hips to support their weight.

Key to correction:

- Lower abdominal musculature and external oblique require strengthening.
- Hip flexors also require strengthening, particularly the iliopsoas which is weak and in an overlengthened position. External rotators of the hip abductors (gluteus medius and tensor fascia latae) and the hip extensors (gluteus maximus) also require strengthening.

Sway back is often associated with a long kyphotic thoracic spine (see kyphosis, page 43 for specific exercises) and a cervical spine lordosis.

Specific exercise: try and soften the hyperextended knees by transferring body weight onto the balls of the feet rather than the heels. Try to think of pulling the chin in, lengthening the back of the neck and lifting the weight up and off your hips. The key to correction is being strong enough in the muscles of the hips, lower back and lower abdominals to lift and maintain the torso up and off the ligaments of the hips.

Military

Key feature: These people give the illusion they have good posture but in fact carry a lot of tension and tightness in their muscles.

Key to correction:

- A general flexibility programme is essential for this postural type. Must include upper and lower back, shoulder, pectorals, hip flexors, hamstrings, adductors, abductors, calves and achilles.
- Strengthening of lower abdominals and external obliques is usually required. Upper abdominals are usually tight and shortened.

Specific exercise: remember you don't need to stand 'at attention' all the time. Try to relax the shoulders particularly while standing, without slumping.

Assessing your postural type

To be sure you have classified yourself correctly as a certain postural type and are doing the right exercises; the following guidelines will give you an idea of what to look for when you are assessing your posture. As mentioned previously you may even have certain aspects of a few of the above postural types.

The ideal way to assess your posture is to take photos from the front, both sides and behind. If you draw a vertical line through the side views you will not only obtain a clearer perspective of your postural type but will also be able to assess more accurately where your body is beginning to give in to gravity. Drawing horizontal lines through the tips of the shoulders, the top of the hips and through the knee-caps will also assist with your postural assessment. On your dominant hand side you will find this shoulder dropped and slightly inwardly rotated and the foot more externally rotated. A slight difference in shoulder height is fine, but greater than 1 centimetre can cause stress in underlying joints. If you have one leg longer than the other, the foot on the longer side will also turn outwards and the knee will hyperextend to accommodate the increased length. Less than 1 centimetre is not considered significant.

Another method that can assist the accuracy of your assessment is using an engineer's flexi-curve to assess the curves in your spine. Place the curve on your spine and mould it to the curves. Then sketch the outline onto paper. Now when you reassess your posture after you have been practising your exercises, see if your spinal curves have altered. Are they closer to the ideal?

Other helpful tools are a carpenter's spirit level, to be more precise when measuring hip and shoulder height. For health professionals, the ideal is to have a postural grid plate.

Aside from the above methods, simple visual assessment using a mirror can indicate clearly to you where muscle imbalance is occurring. A key point to remember is that what you are observing statically is how you use your body dynamically. For instance, if you have a sedentary occupation, and sit hunched over a desk, your static posture will reflect this.

From all four directions, using the three Ts principle will assist your observation. This refers to:

1. **Torsion** — Your neck muscles seem to be twisted one way, or one shoulder appears torsioned and rotated.
2. **Tone** — Some of your muscles look stronger than others, or some look tighter. Compare the size of the quadriceps to the hamstrings. The buttocks appear to be wasted, as usually occurs in flat back or sway back posture.
3. **Tilt** — Your head seems to be to one side. You may have more rolls of fat on one side of your stomach compared with the other.

These three aspects are general considerations. Below are more specific features to look for when you view your body from the front, the side and behind. Remember, posture does reflect how we feel about ourselves and also our emotions, so the features outlined below are a very clinical way of viewing and assessing our body. Nonetheless, if our physical stance is more positive and posture more upright, our mental attitudes and emotions will inherently become more positive.

Observation from the front

What is the ideal from the front?

- Slightly dropped shoulder on the dominant hand side is quite normal.
- There should be no marked hollows above or below the clavicles.
- Marked head tilt may indicate tight neck musculature.
- Hands should lie with palms facing the thighs. Tight shoulder, elbow or weak upper back musculature may prevent this.
- The abdomen should not appear to be sagging.
- A vertical line drawn through the middle of the patellae should drop down and end between the first and second toe. That is, the patellae should be directly over the foot.
- Turnout of the feet less than 30 degrees is within the norm. Less is preferable.

Observation from the side

What is the ideal from the side?

Assess from both sides.

A plumb line should go through the middle of the ear, middle of the shoulder, middle of the femur and run slightly anterior to the lateral malleolus.

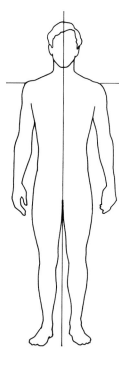

Head tilt

Shoulder height: is it different?

Do the shoulders turn inwards?

Do the muscles around the neck and clavicles look tight?

Are there hollows above or below the collarbones?

Height at the top of the hips

Which way do the patellae point?

Which way are the feet facing: are they the same direction as the patellae?

Do you have inward or outward curves of the femur or tibia?

3.11   Postural assessment from the front

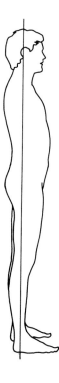

Which postural type?

Is the neck curved inwards indicating tight neck extensors?

How far is the chin forward?

Is the upper part of your spine humped? All of it or just at one place?

Are your abdominal muscles protruding and sagging downwards indicating weak lower abdominal muscles?

Is the curve of your lumbar region too far inwards or is it flat?

Are your buttock muscles strong or do you have no buttock muscles?

Are your knees locked back or slightly bent?

3.12   Postural assessment from the side

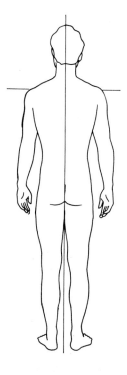

Tilt of the head

Shoulder height

Winged scapula indicating a weakness in shoulder muscles

Stronger muscles on one side of your spine

A side-bent or s-shaped curve in your spine indicating a scoliosis

Hip height uneven

Uneven buttock folds

Uneven creases in the back of your knees

Can you see too much of the front of the foot? This may indicate mid- or forefoot abduction

Are your heels broad and square where your body weight is, or very pointed?   The latter means your weight is on the front of your feet

3.13   Postural assessment from the back

Observation from behind

What is the ideal from the behind?

- Symmetry and balance should exist between the right and left sides of the body, excepting the effects of handedness patterns.
- Heights of the shoulders, the hips, the buttocks etc. should be relatively even.
- Winged scapula indicates imbalance in shoulder muscles, weakness in lower trapezius fibres, usually tightness in the rhomboids, and weakness in the serratus anterior.
- An s-shaped spine is called a scoliosis. This may be structural (you were born with it) or posturally related. When standing and you flex the spine forwards, if the curve disappears it usually indicates the curve is postural and due to some form of muscle tightness, weakness or imbalance. When you bend forwards, if the curve remains, this is called a structural scoliosis. Factors such as a leg length difference may cause or contribute to either of these types of spinal curves. A heel raise provided by a qualified health practitioner can correct spinal imbalance created by length discrepancy. However, stretch-

ing the muscles of the hip and trunk (iliopsoas and quadratus lumborum) can often correct an apparent leg length discrepancy and should be tried first. Other structural curves require specific exercises prescribed by a musculo-skeletal specialist (for instance, a physiotherapist), to prevent long term problems developing.

- Consult a podiatrist if you appear to have flat feet (often called pronated feet) if you have observed this from both the front and from behind, particularly if you have a c-shaped achilles tendon.

CORRECTING YOUR POSTURE

Once you have noted all these independent aspects of your posture, try to create an overall picture of what the balance and symmetry is like in your body. Try to figure out the worst thing you think is happening to your body. This should hope-fully provide you with the key as to where you need to start to correct your posture.

Once you have assessed your posture from the front, both sides and from behind, you should be able to classify yourself as one of the above postural types and design your own daily exercise programme. Chapter 7 lists the exer-cises recommended for each postural type. If you have features of one or more of the types, you will need to extract the most pertinent exercises to suit your specific needs.

Assessing your body dynamically can also help you observe poor postural patterns. Watch yourself walking towards a mirror. Does your body move evenly as you walk? Observing your footprints in the sand on the beach can also tell you a lot about how you distribute your body weight both statically and dynamic-ally. That is, can you notice one foot turns out more than the other? Or if you are flat footed you will see the whole shape of your foot on the sand whereas you should only see the heel, the lateral border of the arch and forefoot.

If you are uncertain about where your postural problems exist, do not hesitate to consult a health professional who specialises in postural assessment. Maybe you have ideal posture — it is possible! If you are an athlete, video analysis can be done to detect the finer points of imbalance that may be taking place in your body while you are exercising.

If you are able to design your own exercise programme, aim for quality move-ments not high-speed, ineffective movements.

Keep in mind that ideal posture includes balance and poise around joints, not just strength and flexibility. Think of the way dancers move their bodies when they walk; almost as though something is lifting them. This is the goal of ideal posture where movement is relaxed, efficient, and a balance between agonist and antagonists at all joints exists.

If you find the suggested exercises unsuitable for your body you may find other methods such as the 'Alexander Technique' or 'Feldenkrais Movement through Awareness Exercises', which are much gentler methods of deprogramming habitual postural patterns, more suited to your needs. The Suggested Reading List provides further details on these methods.

Checklist for good posture

- Postural exercises (as shown in Chapter 7) should be performed daily.
- Make sure your workplace is ergonomically efficient. Your desk and chair should be the right height for you and lighting should be adequate.
- If you play sport, make sure you play a sport suitable to your body type. Invest in the right equipment.
- At home, all benches and worktops should also be the right height. If you are tall you may need to have them altered to suit your specific needs.
- Try not to wear abnormally high heels nor excessively flat shoes with no arch support. Both affect posture adversely, particularly high heels which cause increased stress on the lower back.
- Maintaining a positive outlook on life always helps.

TAPING

Another method that can be used for postural correction is taping. It is best to work with a physiotherapist who specialises in postural correction to assess if you are suited to trying the Taping Technique. However, provided the following precautions are taken, it is fine to try it by yourself.

Taping is a very effective way of reminding the brain and body of what 'normal' and 'ideal' posture is, but if pain is increased by using the tape, it may not be a suitable technique for you.

Taping for postural correction

Uses for taping

- Suitable for correction of kyphotic/lordotic postures.
- May be worn while exercising, or when working in a sedentary occupation.
- Usually not suitable for children under nine or ten years old.
- Ideal for adolescent children during stages of rapid growth.
- May be applied by health professionals or lay people.

Application

Pull the tape firmly across the shoulders while an exaggerated corrected posture is being adopted. Skin layers should not be trapped under the tape.

Procedure

Leave the tape on for one day initially. You may shower while the tape is on. Where possible, postural corrective exercises should be performed within the limitations the tape provides. Repeat two to three days later. Leave on for twenty-four hours if possible. Finally, repeat as you feel necessary to remind yourself how to correct your posture. After three trial sessions results should be observed; if not, an alternative method of correcting posture should be used.

Precautions

If the skin is sensitive, use some form of thin foam underwrap to protect the skin, and only leave the tape on for one hour's trial run.

If a mild increase in mid-thoracic discomfort results during the first twenty-four hours of taping, this is not a cause for concern. Pain for longer than this indicates that taping is not suitable for you.

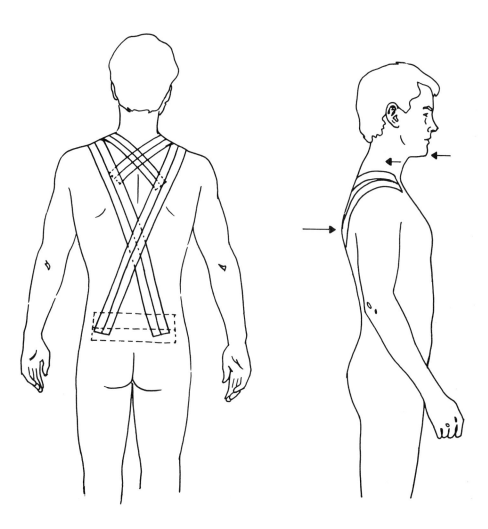

General advice

Encourage pressing the lumbar spine into the tape.

   You will need to cross your legs to put shoes on, also you will need to tighten the buttocks (gluteus maximus) to assist you when you get in and out of chairs.

Tape

Use a good quality flesh coloured sports strapping about 3.5 centimetres wide.

COMMONLY ASKED QUESTIONS

What is the ideal posture for a child?

When a child is just learning to walk, a wide base for the feet and a fairly lordosed lumbar spine is the norm. (See Figure 3.14.) As they get beyond the age of 6 to 11, this marked curve and protruding stomach should become less noticeable. Curved, rounded shoulders with protruding scapulae are not normal for the growing child. It is important to keep an eye on children as they grow as corrective exercises performed in the early years may prevent many problems when they are older. The postural problems children develop are usually related to carrying heavy school bags on one shoulder. It is highly recommended that school satchels carried on the back, distributing the weight through both shoulders, be used in these growing years.

   Stress plays an important part in the development of our posture too. We all experience stress in some form or other, both negatively and positively. It is not so much the stress itself which is harmful, but how we react to it, both physically and mentally.

   Stress causes fatigue of muscles which in turn can lead to the development of poor posture. If you find you suffer too much from stress it is a good idea to join relaxation classes or even to try and learn meditation, or some other form of relaxation, no matter what your age.

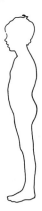

3.14   Normal posture of a child

How long can I expect it to take before I see changes in my posture?

This depends on your age, your height and what your current lifestyle habits are.

If you have noticed your posture getting worse over the last few months or years you will find the results of your exercising will become visible often within the first month or even sooner. Particularly if you have recently changed to sedentary desk work or have just had a baby (especially if you are breast-feeding), your posture may only have deteriorated in the short term. By 6 months you will be able to see if you have retained the changes. If you keep regressing back to your old posture ask yourself what other factors are influential in your daily lifestyle. Maybe you need to look within and ask yourself what is preventing you from projecting a strong and balanced image towards the world — that is to your friends and the community around you.

If you still feel you are unable to achieve changes, make some enquiries about who does postural assessments in your community. Other deep tissue techniques called fascial work, deep connective tissue massage or simply any form of massage, will assist with release of muscles that have been tight for many years. Therapists who do this type of work may be physiotherapists specialised in this area, or others who do rolfing, trager therapy, or hellerwork to mention but a few. (See Suggested Reading List, Rolf, I.)

This type of work may be suitable for you if your posture keeps regressing to its old form.

Can I prevent arthritis by improving my posture?

There are many types of arthritis. Osteoarthritis and rheumatoid arthritis are the two main forms. Osteoarthritis (OA) refers generally to the degeneration or change in the joint surfaces. OA is more marked where weight is not evenly distributed through a particular joint for example, the knees. Research does indicate however that arthritis also tends to occur where nutrition to a joint surface is not good, particularly in non weight-bearing joints (the shoulders) and in joints taking imbalanced load or stress.

While not scientifically or conclusively proven, the implications of these findings would certainly tend to suggest that a person with poor posture is going to be more predisposed to degenerative conditions such as arthritits because of the imbalanced load being taken through their joints. Therefore, exercises to improve posture and which also improve flexibility and balance around a joint, will subsequently decrease abnormal load and stress on the joint, hence decreasing the possibility of arthritis occurring.

Rheumatoid arthritis is not like osteoarthritis. It is a disease which tends to be hereditary and has stages of remission or exacerbation. Exercises may assist when the joints are not in a flared-up stage. Children may get this form of arthritis. This is called juvenile arthritis. Swollen and aching joints throughout the body for no particular reason or injury is the usual presentation. Blood tests can confirm rheumatoid arthritis, while OA joints will show up on x-ray.

4 — EXERCISE, SPORT AND MUSCLES

Now we understand the basic principles of muscle fitness and have designed an exercise programme for improving our posture, we are ready to prepare for our own specific sport. This chapter looks at how to prepare the body for exercise or sport, reviews some basic training tips and discusses how to stay motivated in your fitness programme. Whether you are overtraining is also questioned. Minimal detail to the cardiovascular system and to exercise physiology is covered in *The Muscle Fitness Book*. (Refer to the Suggested Reading List if you wish to understand and study the energy systems utilised for each sport.)

PREPARING FOR SPORT

In cold weather would you turn your car on and drive straight off without giving it any choke? Our body is just like a car. Prior to any sporting activity it needs to be prepared and at the completion it also needs attention. Prior to sport, adequate warm-up can decrease the risk of injury and improve your sporting efficiency, while a cool-down at the completion of your activity can reduce the risk of chronic injuries developing.

Warm-up

This should include a loosening of all the major muscles and limbs in the body, whether they are being used in your particular sport or not. Large circular and swinging movements of the arms and a brisk walk or light jog is a helpful general warm-up. Stretching is also essential for loosening stiff muscles and joints prior to sport. Warm-up, including the stretching, should take a minimum of 10–15 minutes — longer when it is cold.

Cool-down

After sport it is equally important to take a few precautionary measures — particularly to avoid post-exercise muscle soreness. Most sporting activities use some muscle groups more than others. Both these muscles and those that were not necessarily used in the activity must be stretched out at the completion of exercise. This will also reduce your risk of injury next time you exercise. Depending on the intensity of your activity, spend 10–15 minutes cooling down.

TRAINING TIPS

Whatever your sport, it is important to consider all aspects of physical fitness in your preparation and training. Usually these are called the three Ss. These are:

Stamina

This refers to the cardiovascular component of your sport. Are the demands of your sport aerobic or anaerobic or does it combine both? Lack of stamina, particularly in contact sports, can lead to fatigue and an increased risk of injury.

Strength

Does your sport overdevelop the dominant side of your body? If so, you need exercises to balance this effect. Do you have adequate strength for your activity? Maybe an increase in strength would improve your sporting performance.

Suppleness

Regular flexibility exercises are essential to maintain the suppleness in our joints, ligaments and muscles and will enhance sporting performance.

Not only should you attend to each of the above but each sport requires specific skills and these should be practised in training. The following are a few specific training tips:

Change of direction activities

You need to practise agility skills, change of direction activities and stop/start manoeuvres if this is required in your sport. For example, for all codes of football, shuttle sprints gradually increasing the pace and distance, are an ideal form of specific skill training.

Duration and nature of specific skills

You need to practise both physically and mentally (that is, mentally rehearse) the specific skills required in your sport. Do not just practise hard first serves for tennis prior to a match, but aim for accuracy at a slower speed first, then progress to a few harder serves.

Intensity

Try to train at an appropriate intensity for your sport. Do not just do 3 kilometre slow jogs if the fun run you wish to compete in is a 15 kilometre event and you know you will run faster in this than a slow jog pace. Incorporate some longer 10 and 12 kilometre runs in your pre-fun run training.

Range of movement

Ensure you have the full active and passive range of movement for your sport so that other parts of your body are not overloaded. For example, if you are kyphotic and therefore stiff in your thoracic spine, this can limit shoulder movement resulting in shoulder pain if the appropriate corrective exercises are not performed.

Balance, rhythm and timing

Have you practised skills at match pace in training? For example, for basketball have you practised long shot 3 point goals as well as difficult shots under the basket at close range?

Progression

Are you progressing in your training programme gradually? An increase in training pace, distance or intensity too quickly can cause injury.

EXERCISE AND MOTIVATION

Many people take up a fitness programme with zest and enthusiasm but within a few months have abandoned it. The usual reason given is they have lost interest, suffered an injury, are too tired to keep it up or simply do not have time to do the activity regularly.

One of the problems when people take up a fitness programme is that they do not set their goals realistically and they choose activities they feel they *should* do, not what they feel is fun and enjoyable.

When you take up any fitness programme Gary Egger, in his book *The Sport Drug*, proposes three phases you may experience:

1 The discomfort phase

This is in the initial stages when you know you should exercise but your body and mind are telling you differently.

2 The physical phase

This is where you find you can physically exercise more easily. For example, you can go further when you are jogging with greater ease, but your mind still considers the activity a chore.

3 The addicted stage

This is when you cannot go a day without exercising. However, it is possible to be either negatively or positively addicted to exercise. Addiction becomes negative when obsessiveness sets in. At this stage, one day of no exercise will lead to the individual experiencing withdrawal symptoms, such as depression, lethargy, or loss of appetite to mention but a few! Obviously, the ideal is to find the right balance. Regular exercise will enhance one's daily lifestyle, work, home life and so on, but once you start to panic if you miss only one session of your regular exercise, imbalance in the other areas of your life will set in. Therefore, positive addiction in moderation is excellent while negative addiction has potential hazards in all aspects of one's life.

EXERCISE AND MODERATION

Unfortunately, it is possible to exercise too much. With the upsurge of interest in sport this past decade, there has also been a corresponding increase in injuries. Many of these could have been prevented had the necessary precautions been taken, while others are purely related to the fact that people do too much exercise for their bodies to cope with. Injuries falling into this category are called 'overuse injuries'.

How much exercise is enough and how much is too much is not an easy question to answer as every individual and his or her respective needs are different. The answer lies in common sense. If you are waking up each morning feeling tired and exhausted and are having to walk down the stairs backwards because you are too sore to walk straight down, it is highly likely you are overexercising! Unfortunately, for some individuals, their income *is* their exercising so rest is not possible when they get tired or get an injury. Fitness instructors are classic examples of this. Employees and employers should give consideration to this when terms of agreement for employment are being negotiated. Fatigue is a prime precursor to injury for the fitness instructor so common sense should be adhered to for even the smallest injuries, to prevent a chronic problem developing.

COMMONLY ASKED QUESTIONS

Why do I get stiff and sore muscles a few days after exercising?

There are a number of reasons why we get sore muscles when we exercise. One fallacy is that sore muscles are due to lactic acid accumulation. This is not the case. Lactic acid is a waste product produced when we exercise but the body removes this lactic acid. Most of it has been absorbed within 20 minutes post-exercise, and within 2 hours, traces of lactic acid are minimal.
There are four main reasons proposed for muscle soreness:
The pressure theory suggests that post-exercise wastes such as histamines

build up in the muscles and cause, pressure and therefore pain. Weightlifters tend to support this idea but it has little scientific support.

The spasm theory claims that ischaemia (pooling of blood), caused by exercise, results in the production of a pain substance (substance P) which in turn causes further pain. The evidence supporting this idea remains contradictory.

The tear theory proposes that pain is caused by microtears in muscle fibres following unaccustomed movement. Examination for chemicals in exercised muscles, which could be indicative of tears, however, has shown that these exist independently of pain.

The connective tissue theory is perhaps the most scientifically supported theory of muscle pain. This is based on observations that soreness is most common following negative (eccentric) muscle contractions, rather than following positive (concentric) muscle contractions. Research indicates that negative contractions put a greater strain on a muscle's non-contractile components (the connective tissue). This is supported by the observation that soreness is usually located in and around the tendon of an eccentrically contracted muscle. Microtears in the connective tissue, as opposed to the contractile muscle fibres, are thought to cause the pain.

None of these reasons has been conclusively proven but the most scientifically accepted one is the connective tissue theory. It is important to note here that stretching prior to, and at the completion of, exercises reduces post-exercise soreness, particularly when the exercise is not familiar. This tends to be when muscle soreness occurs most often.

Why do I weigh more when I take up a fitness programme when I am trying to lose weight?

This aspect of muscle fitness often causes great concern for those who take up an exercise programme to lose weight. However, the explanation for this phenomenon is really quite simple. Basically, muscle weighs more than fat. Therefore, as we get fitter, we usually develop our muscles, and if our programme is aerobic we will probably lose overall body fat content. But if we stand on our scales we will therefore weigh more. This is why scales are not a very accurate measure of our true weight as they do not take into account muscle size.

If we carry fat deposits on specific areas of our body, is it possible to spot reduce?

The answer to this is definitely, no. By exercising a specific muscle we can increase its tone and strength but the only way to lose fat from a specific area is to participate in aerobic exercise regularly and to reduce overall body fat content. So if you have a very large protruding stomach, sit-ups will not reduce its size, but purely give you a firm strong stomach! (Aerobic exercise would be highly recommended in this instance.) As mentioned previously, hormonal and postural factors do influence where we deposit some of the fat in our body.

Why do we tend to bulk in some muscles and not others when we do weight training?

This is a very interesting phenomenon. Why do the abdominal or stomach muscles not bulk in size as much as our biceps for instance? Why do the back muscles not bulk up as much as the quadriceps?

These are fascinating questions, but as yet the answers are unclear. Scientific research tends to indicate that these size differences are more neurologically predetermined as opposed to differences in the type of muscle cell or fibre present in different areas of the body.

The most visible differences that occur in weight training are the size increases to the peripheral muscles — biceps, triceps, deltoid, calves, quadriceps and hamstrings.

The muscles of the trunk — the abdominals, back extensors, the hip flexors (iliopsoas), tend not to bulk so readily.

The only plausible explanation at this stage appears to be related to the relative composition of individual muscles and also their functional demands. Back extensors and stomach muscles tend to be more fibritic in nature. That is, they have a higher component of connective tissue. Connective tissue is denser, stronger and provides more stability and strength than do the contractile components of the muscle. Back extensors are working continuously to support our posture while the abdominal muscles (all four) support and retain our abdominal and pelvic structures. Alternatively, muscles that contribute more significantly to peripheral joints (biceps, triceps and gastrocnemius, for instance) tend to have a larger muscle belly and contain relatively less connective tissue. This difference in composition may be why these peripheral muscles can bulk more readily than trunk muscles, which do increase markedly in strength with exercise, but not necessarily size. Also, the contractile components of a muscle have the ability to increase in size (called hypertrophy of a muscle), whereas overload on the connective tissue does not have this same effect.

It must be noted though that this explanation is purely hypothetical at this stage and scientific explanations for this phenomenon are as yet unknown.

Are there any other facts and fallacies regarding muscles and exercise I should know?

The main areas where fact and fallacy are often difficult to discern, is with respect to weight loss and muscles. The following comments attempt to dispel some of these myths.

- Vibrator belts and cellulite wraps *do not* help you to lose fat. Vibrators may provide a little massage and may relax tight muscles, which can certainly cause no harm, but certainly do not rub away fat.
- Saunas do not help one lose weight. After a sauna, scales may indicate you weigh less but this is purely due to fluid loss. This effect is negated once you increase your fluid intake again.

- Contrary to popular belief, fat does not turn to muscle when you exercise making it ineffective to spot reduce. Fat can only be reduced by aerobic exercise or reducing kilojoule intake in your diet, such that energy expenditure is greater than the energy taken in by food. However, the reduction in your food intake should not be excessive or your body learns to adjust to the minimal intake. Specific exercise for a particular area of the body will tone a muscle but not necessarily utilise the fat in this particular area.
- Women will not bulk if they use weights. Muscle bulk is determined largely through the involvement of the male hormone testosterone. While this hormone does exist in females it is usually not in sufficient quantities to allow muscle bulking. Strength and body shaping exercises will assist in decreasing body fat and improving muscle tone, but will not cause bulking unless synthetic hormones such as anabolic steroids are used.

PART 2 — THE EXERCISES

5 — EXERCISES FOR EACH PART OF THE BODY

This chapter outlines exercises to stretch and strengthen each part of the body. Exercises for correcting posture are also taken from this list of exercises. Both stretching and strengthening exercises are outlined for all the major muscles and muscle groups of the body, starting with the cervical spine or neck, working down to the shoulders, then the trunk (which includes the abdomen and the back) and finally the lower limb, which includes the hips, thighs, calves and feet.

In the following chapters, Daily routines, Exercises for special groups, and Exercises for specific sports, the most appropriate exercises will be extracted and suggested.

STRETCHES AND STRENGTHENING AND MOBILITY EXERCISES

Stretches will improve your flexibility and when you perform them, you should feel the muscle or muscles being stretched. If you cannot feel it, you may not be doing the exercise correctly or it may be an inappropriate exercise for you.

Strengthening is important to provide stability around all joints. You should be aware and feel the muscle you are strengthening. You should not perform the exercise so quickly that you are using momentum to achieve the movement as opposed to specifically strengthening a particular muscle.

Both stretching and strengthening are important to achieve balance around our joints. No individual muscle should be stretched excessively or laxity about a joint on one side will result. Do not avoid the exercises that are difficult to do as these are usually the ones you need most!

If an exercise is working a particular muscle, this is stated; many of the exercises are a combination of movements, however, involving a few muscles. The shading on some stretches indicates where you should feel the exercise. The arrows indicate the direction in which you should move your body.

Stretches

Hold all stretches for 6–10 seconds at a minimum. Relax and breathe out as you move into the stretch. Do not ease back too far before repeating the stretch.

Repeat a minimum of three times. For tighter muscles try to hold the stretch for longer.

Push to the point of discomfort but do not push through pain. *No exercise should produce pain.*

Strengthening exercises

Start with four to six repetitions (less will be noted in parentheses if this is necessary). Progress to eight to ten repetitions. When this becomes too easy, do three sets or use an elastic band or weight to increase the effectiveness of the exercise. Remember quality movement will achieve far more than exercise performed with poor form in large quantities or at high speed.

Mobility exercises

Some exercises combine stretching and strengthening throughout the range. Start with two to three repetitions of these exercises and progress to four to six. All mobility exercises should be taken to as full a range as your body permits. You should feel where they are working.

Neck (×2–3)

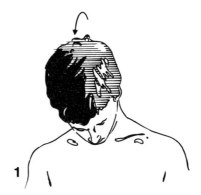

1. **Neck flexion** — to stretch neck extensors. Tuck the chin in and bend the head forward. Relax the shoulders.

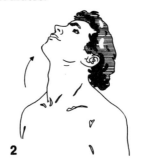

2. **Neck extension** — to stretch neck flexors. Look to the ceiling and stretch the neck back.

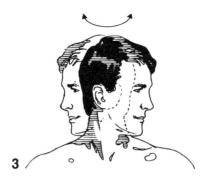

3. **Neck rotation.** Look over one shoulder then the other. Do not let the opposite shoulder come forward. Tuck the chin in.

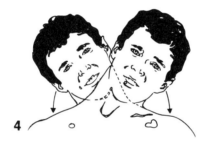

4. **Neck side flexion.** Pull the ear down to the shoulder. Do not let the opposite shoulder raise up.

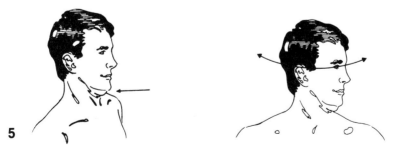

5. **Neck stretch** — to correct a lordotic cervical spine (×2–3). Pull the chin inwards. Create a double chin and gently look to the right, then the left. You should feel the stretch at the side of the neck. Pull the shoulders down gently to increase the effectiveness of the stretch.

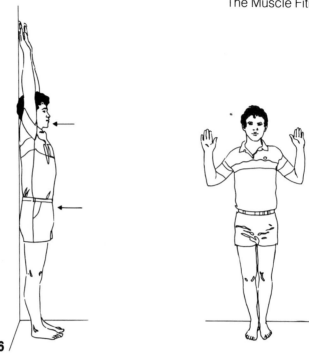

6

6. **Wall exercise** — to correct a cervical spine lordosis and strengthen lower trapezius (standing). If your neck and upper shoulders curve forward this is an excellent exercise for correcting this. It is also ideal for lordosis and kyphosis type postures. Firstly, flatten your back against a wall, with your heels 7–15 centimetres away from the wall. When you start, your feet may need to be further away. As you improve you can place a book in the small of your back as you do the exercise. Now turn the shoulders and thumbs inwards and raise your arms above your head while maintaining a flat back. Breathe in as you initiate the exercise, and exhale as the arms are raised. This exercise strengthens the lower fibres of the trapezius muscle which is always weak in a stooped forward posture.

Now keeping the thoracic spine against the wall, bend your elbows and slide your arms downwards, then stretch up again. Repeat six to eight times daily and you will notice an improvement in your posture within a very short time.

Now repeat this exercise with the hands turned outwards.

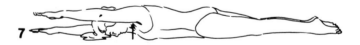

7

7. **Neck extensor and upper back strengthening** — to correct cervical lordosis and thoracic kyphosis. Lying prone, place hands outstretched above the head. Tuck the chin in and lift the head. Keep it in the horizontal plane. Now lift one arm, then the other, by pulling the shoulder blade back to the spine. Do not rotate the torso and keep the elbow close to the ear.

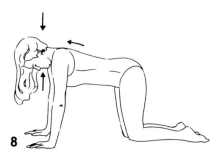

8. Neck stretch and strengthening exercise while on all fours. Alternatively, exercise 7 can be performed on your hands and knees. Keeping the spine straight, create a double chin and elongate the back of the neck. Do not let the shoulders become rounded. This exercise can assist stretching and strengthening the neck extensors which become shortened with poor posture when the chin is thrust forward.

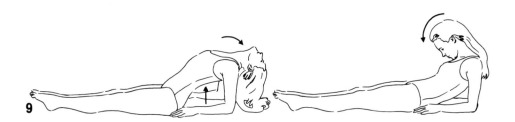

9. Advanced neck strengthening exercise — not recommended if you have neck and/or back pain. Sitting with your legs stretched out and resting on the elbows, gently and very slowly let the head drop backwards. Let the chest pull towards the ceiling. Now very slowly, let the chin and head come forward onto the chest, as the spine curves forward. You must have full pain-free range of movement before trying this exercise.

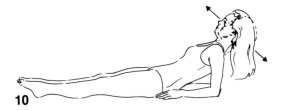

10. For neck mobility and strength — not advisable for those with cervical lordosis. Starting in the same position as for exercise 9, slowly lift the head directly upwards from the body and then let it come back down to create a double chin.

Chest

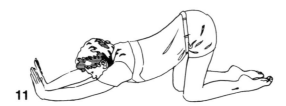

11

11. **Pectoral stretch** — excellent for correcting thoracic spine kyphosis and for tight shoulders. On all fours, place the hands with extended wrists out in front, pull the shoulder blades together and let the thoracic spine drop inwards. Keep the hips directly over the knees. Knees should not be touching.

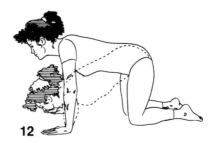

12

12. **Pectoral and tricep strengthening** — modified push-up, variation I. Using a modified push-up position, with elbows kept close to the sides of the body, hands directly under the shoulders, lower and raise the torso, keeping the head and trunk in a straight line.

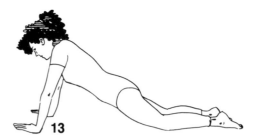

13

13. **Shoulder girdle strengthening** — pectoral, deltoid, triceps, trapezius and rhomboid strengthening, modified push-up, variation II. Using the modified push-up position again, as for exercise 12, place the hands wider than shoulder width. Progress to placing the hands further forward to make the push-up harder, but do not let the back collapse inwards as you are doing the push-up.

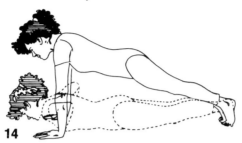

14. **Full push-up** — shoulder and upper back strengthening. Progress to a full push-up if you are able, and place the hands on top of each other to increase the difficulty of the work on the shoulder muscles. Repeat using the hand position of exercises 12 and 13 while doing a full push-up.

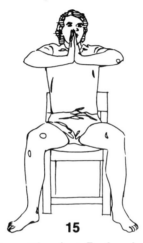

15. **Isometric pectoral strengthening.** Push palms together. You should feel it in your chest muscles. Repeat with arms outstretched above the head.

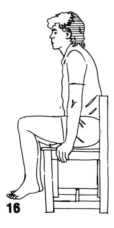

16. **Sitting pectoral and shoulder strengthening.** While sitting on a chair, place hands on either side of the chair, grip, and lift the body weight.

Shoulders and arms

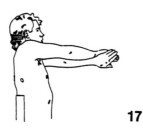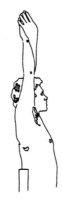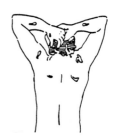

17

17. **Thoracic spine and shoulder mobility exercise** ($\times 4-5$). Cross the arms and clasp hands in front of the body at shoulder height. Take a breath in and as you exhale, stretch the hands above the head. As you again breathe in, bend the elbows and bring the hands down behind the neck. Release the hands so that just the fingers are clasping when the hands are behind the neck. Stretch the arms up again, then repeat, bringing the elbows down again, fingers behind the neck. This is an excellent exercise for reducing stiffness in the shoulders and thoracic spine.

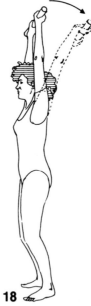

18

18. **Thoracic spine and shoulder mobility exercise using a rod.** Take a rod and clasp it with the palms turned down. Take a breath in as you raise the bar up, and then breathe out as you slowly ease the bar over and behind the body. Keep a wide grip initially and do not force the bar backwards. Aim to achieve the exercise with the hands placed at shoulder width. Do not arch the back and keep the knees slightly flexed. Do not do this exercise if you have shoulders which sublux easily.

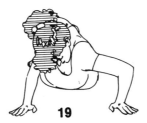

19. **Shoulder and scapula mobility.** Passively arch back from the lower back, keeping the pelvis on the ground. Rotate the shoulder downwards to the floor by letting the elbow come outwards. Think of pulling the scapula away from the spine. Keep the head facing the floor. Do not rotate the lower or mid-back. Excellent stretch for anterior aspect of the shoulder. Not recommended if you have shoulders that sublux or dislocate easily.

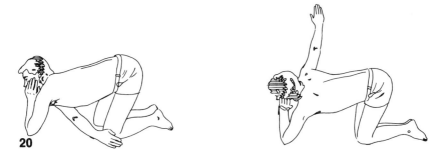

20. **Shoulder and thoracic spine mobility** — for stretching and strengthening the rhomboids as well as for improving general shoulder, scapula and thoracic spine mobility. On all fours, with the chin resting on one hand with the elbow bent, weave one arm through and stretch as far down as possible on the outside of the opposite leg. Counter-resist here to stretch the rhomboids. Now rotate from the mid-back and pull the arm back up and behind.

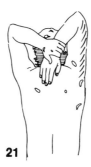

21. **Tricep stretch.** Hand up and behind the neck, resist against the other hand which is placed on the back of the wrist. Point the elbow to the ceiling.

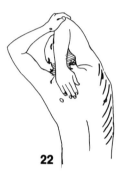

22. **Latissimus dorsi stretch.** Place one hand up and behind the neck. Bring the other hand up and onto the outside of the elbow. Gently pull it down. Increase the stretch by side-bending to the side opposite to the arm you are stretching.

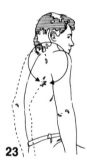

23. **Shoulder rotations: sitting** — for shoulder mobility. Rotate each shoulder forward, up, and back. Do not move the chest upwards. Keep the spine straight. Now rotate the shoulders in the opposite direction.

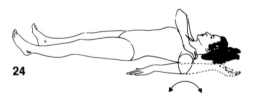

24. **Shoulder rotation lying on your back** — pectoralis major and minor stretch. Place one arm with bent elbow at right angles to the body. Place the other hand on top of the shoulder. Rotate the hand and forearm upwards and forwards to the floor. Do not let the shoulder roll upwards or forwards as the hand is moved.

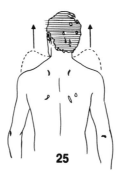

25. **Shoulder shrugs** — for shoulder mobility. Lift both shoulders up to the ears. Tighten then release, then let them relax again. Do not poke the chin forward as you do this. An ideal exercise if you are a student or have a sedentary occupation.

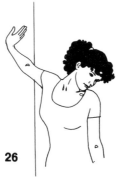

26. **Wrist, shoulder and neck stretch.** Side-tilt the head away from the arm being stretched, then take this arm behind and pull the fingers onto the back of the wrist. Use a wall or door to resist against. A helpful exercise if you get pain in your forearm referring from your neck, though do not do it if your pain is aggravated.

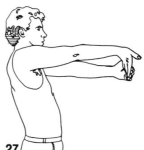

27. **Wrist and finger stretch.** With arms outstretched, pull the fingers back towards the forearm. Repeat by stretching the fingers in the opposite direction onto the back of the wrist. Vary the angle of your hand so you are stretching more effectively.

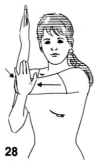

28

28. **Thoracic spine and rhomboids stretch.** One arm bent at right angles, held at horizontal level. Place the back of the hand at the back of the elbow. Counter-resist at this point. Resist then pull it across the body further. You should feel the stretch between the shoulder blades. Vary the height of your arms if you cannot feel any stretch.

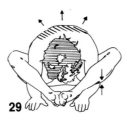

29

29. **Upper back stretch** — rhomboids and posterior shoulder stretch. Sit with the soles of your feet together. Place the hands under the ankles and put the palms on the floor. Push down with the ankles. Pull up between the shoulder blades. Aim to place the elbows on the floor and try to think of the top of the head touching the floor as you are relaxing forward. Slowly move the hands forward, away from the body, and bring the heels closer to the body to increase the effectiveness of the stretch. If you cannot tuck your hands under the ankles, and have your elbows on the floor, do not attempt to do this exercise and replace it with exercise 28.

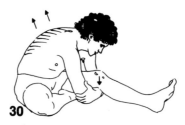

30

30. **Posterior shoulder and thoracic spine stretch** — sitting. Tuck the hands or cross the arms under one knee. Tuck the chin in. Pull up in between the shoulder blades as you try to straighten the knee. Not recommended if you have back pain.

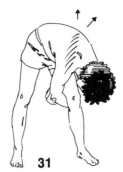

31. **Posterior shoulder and upper back stretch** — standing. While standing with legs comfortably apart, bend one knee, then clasp the arms or elbows around it. Straighten the knee as you pull up between the shoulder blades. Progress to doing exercise with feet together if you are flexible enough. Not recommended if you have back pain.

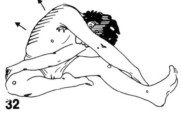

32. **Latissimus dorsi/quadratus lumborum stretch.** Sitting, one leg bent, with the foot just resting against the inside of the opposite thigh, place the opposite hand on this leg then bring the other hand over and reach towards the outstretched leg. If you can clasp the outside of the ankle, look under the elbow and pull up to stretch the side of the trunk. If you cannot reach the outstretched leg, replace this with exercise 33.

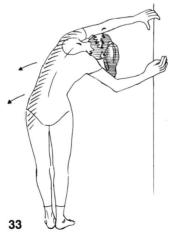

33. **Side trunk stretch.** This stretch can be done by standing adjacent to a wall. Keep the feet parallel to the wall and let the body lean outwards, away from the wall.

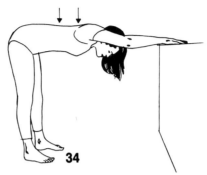

34. **Advanced thoracic spine mobility.** Place both hands on a table at hip height. Aim to pull the shoulder blades together and curve the thoracic spine inwards. You can bend the knees if the hamstrings are tight. Excellent for thoracic kyphosis. Progress to elbows on the table with the hands placed behind the neck, when increased flexibility of the shoulders is gained.

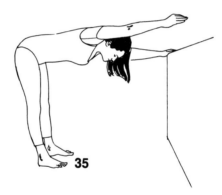

35. **Upper back strengthening** — for rhomboids, trapezius and back extensors. Hands on table at hip height. Keep the elbow close to the ear. Do not rotate the trunk. Raise the arm (this strengthens the rhomboids and upper back extensors). Keep the elbow close to the ear. If your hamstrings are tight, you may need to bend the knees.

Back

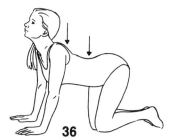

36

36. **Cat stretch** — mobility exercise for the spine: extension. Breathe in as you let the spine curve inwards, pull the shoulder blades together. Keep the knees directly under the hips. Breathe out as you curve upwards. Move gently up then down. Do not hold each position. *Caution* — if you have a back complaint do not let the back drop down past the horizontal.

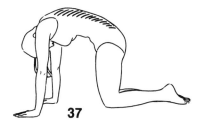

37

37. **Cat stretch** — mobility exercise for the spine: flexion. See exercise 36.

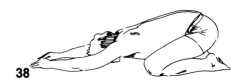

38. **Lower back release** — relaxation position (×1 — hold 20–30 seconds).
Gently try to place the lower back and buttocks between the feet. Be sure to
have the tops of the feet touching the floor.

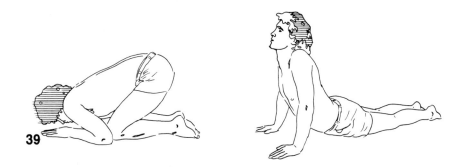

39. **Spinal flexion/extension stretch.** After cat stretch and lower back release keep the chin close to the floor. Follow closely to the floor and move into
an arched back position. You may need to move the hands forward a little before
commencing the second part of this stretch.

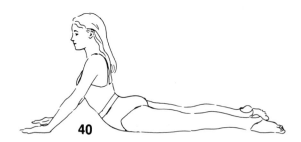

40. **Passive back extension stretch** (×4–5). Keeping the hands under the
shoulders and trying to keep the pelvis on the floor, pull the shoulder blades
together and let the back muscles relax as you arch back. Caution — do not do
this exercise if your back aches when you lie prone (i.e., when you lie on your
abdomen).

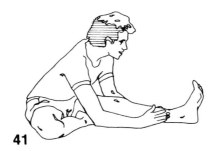

41

41. **Lower back stretch.** Outstretch one leg and keep the other leg bent. Keep hands or elbows on the floor if you can, and gently keep moving forward. Hold each position for 6–10 seconds before you stretch forwards. To increase the effectiveness of the stretch, bring the toes back into a flexed position. Try to move forward from the lumbar, not simply the thoracic spine, which is often already too flexible. Not recommended if you have a kyphotic thoracic spine.

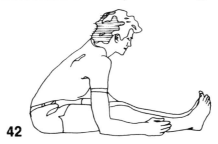

42

42. **Advanced lower back stretch.** See exercise 41. Progress to both legs straight, toes back towards you. Gently curve outwards then inwards in the lower back as you ease forward to increase the effectiveness of the stretch. Keep the hands placed on the floor to take the pressure off the lumbar spine. Do not do this exercise if you only curve forward at the mid- and upper-back.

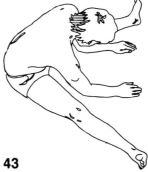

43

43. **Advanced lower back stretch with hip rotation.** See exercises 41 and 42. Progress to legs astride and gently ease forwards using the elbows for support. Only recommended for those who are very flexible. Keep the back straight as you lean forward.

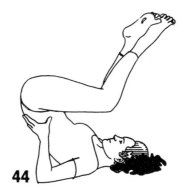

44. Spinal stretch and abdominals strengthening — with bent legs. Gently roll the legs over the head. Support the hips as you do this. Now very slowly unwind the spine, placing each vertebra on the ground individually. Try not to use the hands on the hips, but place them on the floor as you unwind. Control with the abdominal muscles and keep the legs close to the body. Finish off with spinal release (exercise 47). For the bent-leg version of this exercise, cross the ankles, keep the knees turned outward and close to the body, as you roll downwards to starting position.

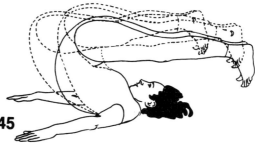

45. Advanced spinal stretch and abdominals strengthening — with straight legs. Use the hands for support as you roll over and use the abdominals as you unwind. Advance by placing the hands on the floor as you unwind. Push the heels together, flex the ankle, do not point. *Caution* — do not perform this exercise if you suffer back pain. Exercises 44 and 45 should never be used in an aerobics class or at high speed. Two to three repetitions is sufficient to obtain benefit from these exercises.

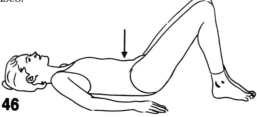

46. Lower back release (×6–8). Lying on the back with knees bent, feet on the floor, press the small of the lower back into the floor. Hold 6–10 seconds, then relax. This is a gentle exercise for easing lower back discomfort.

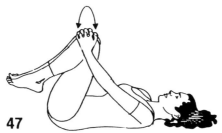

47

47. **Spinal release stretch.** Hands resting on the knees, lift them off the floor. Have the hips at right angles and rotate them to the right then the left, slowly and gently. Keep the knees slightly apart in line with the hips.

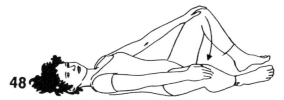

48

48. **Pelvis and lower back release.** Hands resting on top of the knees with feet off the floor, let one leg drop slowly outwards, just short of the floor. Let the other one come over to meet it. Lift the top leg up and over to the other side and repeat. Be gentle and let the exercise flow.

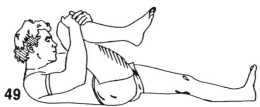

49

49. **Knee hug stretch** — for the hip, gluteus maximus and lower back. Hug one knee up onto the chest. Progress to bringing the forehead to the knee. Advance by keeping the outstretched leg off the ground as you stretch each leg. This will strengthen the abdominals as you stretch the hip extensors.

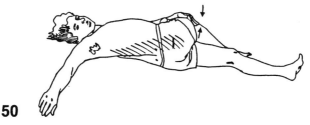

50

50. **Spinal rotation stretch: lying.** Raise one leg up and over the other one. Place the opposite hand on top of the knee. Gently press it to the floor as you keep the other shoulder on the floor, arm outstretched. Look in the direction of the outstretched hand. Progress to straightening the leg. Increase the effectiveness of the stretch by counter-resisting the knee against the hand.

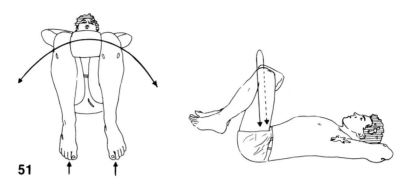

51. **Double leg spinal rotation.** Spinal rotation can also be done with both knees bent up with a rolled towel held between the knees. Rotate both legs one way and then the other.

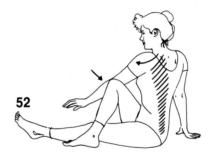

52. **Spinal rotation stretch: sitting.** Place one foot on the outside of the other knee. Rotate the shoulders past the knee. Gently press the elbow against the bent knee. Resist and repeat. Rotate a little further, keeping the spine upright.

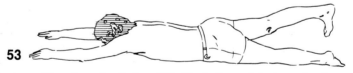

53. **Back strengthening single leg lift.** Push the pelvis into the floor and use the buttock to lift the leg. Try not to arch the lower back. Only lift the leg 15–20 centimetres. Keep the ankle flexed.

54. **Back strengthening single arm lift**. Lift the arm. Keep the elbow close to the ear. (See exercise 7.)

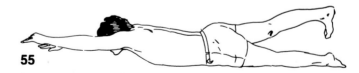

55. **Opposite leg and arm lift strengthening.** Stretch them out long, rather than arching too far. Repeat both sides.

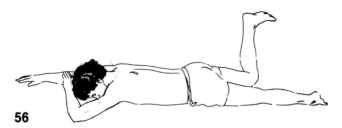

56. **Alternate swimming** — for back strengthening. Try not to arch while bending the opposite foot and arm back towards the head. Repeat each side.

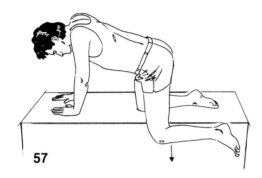

57. **Sacro-iliac joint strengthening.** Resting on all fours near the edge of a table (be sure it is stable before attempting this exercise), let one knee gently lower 8–15 centimetres over the edge of the table. (Using a large book such as a telephone book may be more suitable for you.) Keep the knee and hip at right angles. Now raise this hip and knee vertically, then let them drop again. Repeat. Progress to outstretching the leg closest to the edge of the table behind, at the same time as the opposite arm is outstretched. Now bring the knee and elbow into the chest and hug them together. Then outstretch them again. The first part of this exercise strengthens the sacro-iliac joint that is on the table. The latter part provides balance and control around the joint.

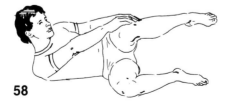

58. **Side-trunk strengthening** — for quadratus lumborum. Lying on your side with both legs at right angles to the body, lift the head and shoulders off the floor at the same time as you lift the top leg. Try to get the hands to the top of the leg. Keep the knee and ankle parallel to the floor.

Hips

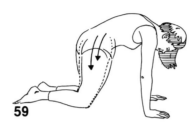

59. **Hip stretch** — for piriformis and sciatica. In cat stretch position, push into one buttock, feel the muscles in the buttock give, then stretch a little further into the hip.

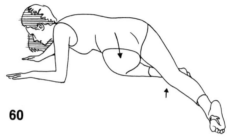

60. **Advanced hip stretch.** In cat stretch position, place one leg at 45 degrees to the body over and behind the other leg. Place the top of this foot to the floor. Let body weight gently stretch into the hip of the bent leg. Do not just collapse to the floor. This stretch will be ineffective for you if you are very flexible.

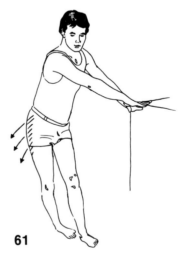

61. **Hip abductor stretch** — tensor fascia latae and iliotibial band. Place the leg to be stretched behind with toes 8–10 centimetres away from the opposite heel. Turn the toes of the behind leg inwards 30 degrees and let body weight fall into this hip. You may need to rest on the heels to get a more effective stretch. Try to rest back and across into the ball and socket joint of the hip.

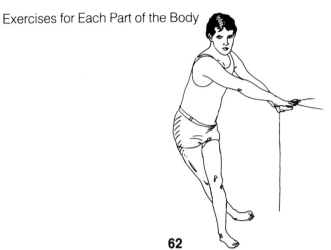

62

62. **Advanced hip abductor stretch.** See above exercise. Now let the leg being stretched come right across the body and let body weight stretch into this leg. Do not side-flex the trunk or you will only be stretching these side muscles as opposed to specifically stretching the muscles in the hip. Always combine this exercise with strengthening of the lateral rotators of the hip (exercise 64) so that you do not overstretch these hip muscles causing an internally rotated femur. Knee problems can occur if the lateral hip rotators are overstretched.

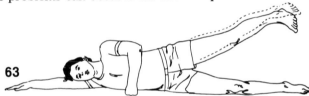

63

63. **Hip strengthening** — gluteus medius and tensor fascia latae. Lying on your side, outstretched. Raise the top leg, keep the toe flexed and turned towards the floor. Lift 25–30 degrees then turn the knee-cap facing straight ahead and lower your leg. Try not to let the legs touch. Do not arch the back and do not tilt the pelvis. Use resistance in this exercise by using a rubber band around the ankles.

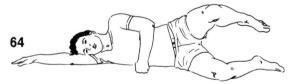

64

64. **Lateral rotators strengthening** — for the hip. Exercise 63 may be done with the top leg bent. This time keep the bottom leg up, flexed 90 degrees at the hip. Keep the body and torso (particularly the hip) in a straight line. Do not arch the back or hyperextend the hip. Raise the top leg, knee bent and slightly higher than the foot. You may need to put a pillow between your knees if this is too difficult initially and raise the top leg just a little off the pillow. Be careful not to flex at the hips. Keep the hips in line with the body. Repeat by raising the leg 10–15 centimetres above hip height and lower the leg slightly below the hip. Keep the knee pointed upwards throughout the exercise.

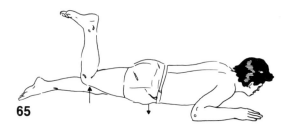

65

65. **Buttock strengthening** — gluteus maximus. Lying prone, bend one leg at right angles, push the pelvis into the floor, tighten the buttock and lift the bent leg. Keep the toe flexed and do not arch the back. This exercise can also be performed when on all fours, that is, in the hands and knees position. Rest on the elbows and do not hyperextend the lower back if trying the exercise this way.

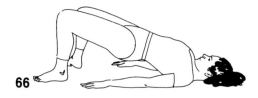

66

66. **Pelvic lift** — gluteus maximus strengthening. Lying on the back, knees bent, feet on the floor, tighten the buttocks and lift the pelvis. Do not arch the back inwards. Maintain the body in a straight plane.

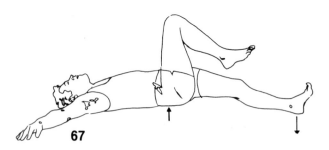

67

67. **Advanced upper hamstring and buttock strengthening.** Lying on the back, one knee bent, other heel on the floor. Tighten the buttocks and raise the pelvis off the floor. Use the heel to push down into the floor.

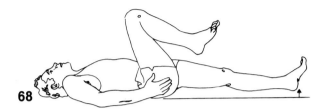

68. **Alternate cycling** — for stabilising hips. Lying on the back, both legs bent up at right angles to the floor. Lift one knee straight upwards, then the other, keep the stomach tight and do not arch the back. (See exercise 73.) Now place the hands on the buttocks and use this muscle, by keeping it tight, to outstretch the leg with toes flexed. Alternate each leg. An excellent exercise for establishing control in the pelvis, particularly for sway back posture. If the back arches before the leg is straight, meaning iliopsoas is stronger than the lower abdominals, bend the knee and start the exercise again. Only take the leg out as far as can be controlled by the abdominals. If you are hypermobile keep your hand on the bony prominence on the outside of the upper thigh (called the greater trochanter) and tighten the buttocks as you extend the leg. This will ensure the femur does not slide upwards which means the hip is rotating inwards, and not extending with control, which is what you want.

Abdomen

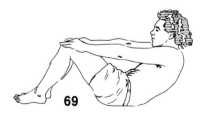

69. **Sit-ups** — upper abdominals strengthening. Not recommended if you have a thoracic kyphosis. With knees bent up, tuck the chin onto the chest and raise the head and shoulders not more than 30 degrees. Tighten the buttocks while you are raising the head and shoulders. Be careful not to poke the chin out and try to keep the head in line with the body as you lift up. Create a double chin before lifting the head and shoulders.

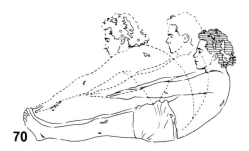

70

70. **Straight leg sit-up** — upper abdominals strengthening. Not recommended if you have a back complaint and not to be done at high speed (i.e., *do not use in aerobics classes*). Ideal for fit dancers, gymnasts and for martial arts experts. The exercise will only hurt your back if you let the lower back arch inwards as you do it. Lying supine, push the back of the knees into a towel rolled under the knees and raise head and shoulders with arms outstretched to 45 degrees. Progress to 90 degrees if this is too easy. Try to curl upwards from each vertebra. Advance to crossing the arms on the chest then to placing the hands on the head and come up as far as you can. If the feet lift off the floor as you raise the head and shoulders, the exercise is too advanced for you. Return to exercise 69.

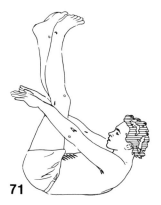

71

71. **Abdominals crunch** — upper abdominal strengthening. Lying on the back, knees raised at right angles to the body and ankles crossed, raise the arms, head and shoulders up 30 degrees to meet the ankles.

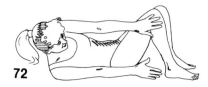

72

72. **Oblique sit-ups** — for external and internal oblique strengthening. Curl the trunk upwards but stretch the hands past the opposite knee. Keep the buttocks tight as you lift.

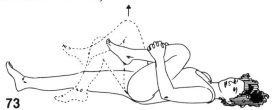

73. **Beginners' lower abdominals strengthening.** Lying on the back, hug one knee onto the chest. Now brace the abdominals (do not just fill the abdomen with air by holding your breath) and raise the opposite leg, keeping the knee at a fixed angle off the floor. You may need to simulate a cough to locate the lower abdominals. Keep one hand on the abdomen to ensure this muscle works throughout the exercise. Now keeping the back on the floor, straighten this leg, then bend up again. Initially, you may need to slide the heel on the floor until you can do the exercise with the leg in the air. If this exercise is too easy progress to exercise 74.

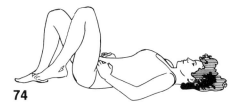

74. **Intermediate lower abdominals strengthening.** Lying on the back, place the hands on the lower abdominals, just inside the hip bone. Tighten and brace. Now lift one knee straight upwards (not towards the chest). Lift the other leg. Try to lift both for 4–6 seconds then relax. If it is too easy you are probably bringing the knee towards the chest, not lifting it 5–8 centimetres towards the ceiling.

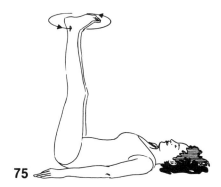

75. **Advanced lower abdominals strengthening.** Raise both legs at right angles to the body. Bend the knees and hips first before you extend the legs. Roll the knees up first — do not do straight leg raise to get the legs in the air. If you cannot keep the knees straight then do not do this exercise. Push the heels together and flex the ankles. Make eight to ten small circles clockwise (only 10–12 centimetres each direction), then repeat anti-clockwise.

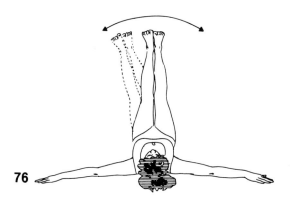

76. Advanced oblique strengthening. Progress to letting the legs drop slowly 20–25 centimetres to each side. Use the opposite abdominals (tighten them) to bring the legs slowly back to the mid-line. Now progress to trying to lift the legs vertically to the ceiling. Keep the toes flexed and the heels pushed together.

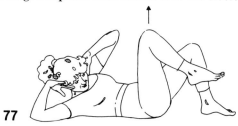

77. Combination oblique strengthening. Knees bent up, raise one knee upwards not towards the chest. Keep the hand beside the head, not under it, with elbow bent. Try to bring the elbow to the knee, not the knee to the elbow.

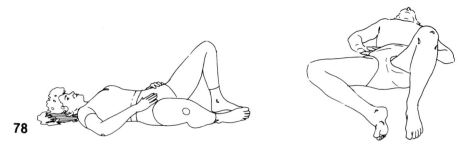

78. Adductor stretch and oblique strengthening. Lying supine, both knees bent up, feet on the floor, place the hands on the inside of the hip bone (on external oblique) then let the knee drop outwards to the floor. Use the obliques on the opposite side to bring the knee back to the mid-line by tightening and bracing the abdomen. Do not let the abdomen protrude outwards. Your bracing should have the effect of pulling the abdomen in and flattening the stomach.

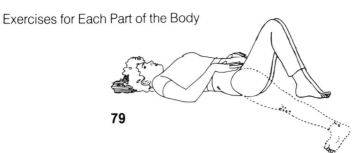

79

79. **Advanced adductor stretch and oblique strengthening.** Progress to doing the exercise with an outstretched leg. Do not let the pelvis roll as the leg drops outwards. Keep it stable and do not arch the back. An ideal exercise for relieving an acute lower back muscle spasm or if you get groin pain.

Thighs

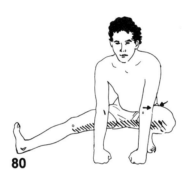

80

80. **Adductor stretch: standing/squatting.** Stand with feet astride, parallel to each other. Now transfer your weight onto one leg and feel the stretch on the inside of the thigh. Repeat by turning the feet out 30–40 degrees and drop the buttocks closer to the floor if you can. Do not do this exercise in the full squat position if it hurts your knees. Keep the elbow on the inside of the bent knee and turn this hip out further to increase the effectiveness of the stretch. Counter-resist at the elbow and knee.

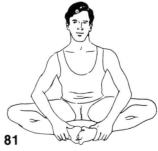

81

81. **Adductor stretch: sitting.** Sitting with soles of feet together, and with the elbows resting on the inside of the knees. Gently counter-resist on the knees, then relax and let the legs stretch closer to the floor.

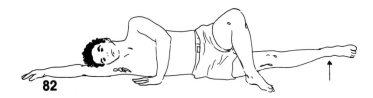

82

82. **Adductor strengthening.** Lying on one side, with top leg bent up and over the other, raise the bottom leg and repeat. Keep the foot of the outstretched leg parallel to the floor. Start with head and shoulders on the floor. Progress to lifting the head up slightly, letting it rest on the hand.

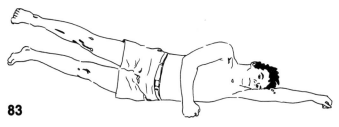

83

83. **Advanced adductor strengthening.** Lying on the side, top leg in the air, lift the bottom leg to meet it. Keep the spine straight. Lower the bottom leg. Do not let it touch the ground. Lift it again and repeat.

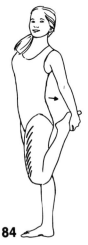

84

84. **Quadriceps stretch.** Clasp the foot first with one, then repeat with the other hand, and pull it towards the buttocks. Keep knees close together. Do not arch the back or flex the hip. Tilt the pelvis posteriorly and shift the front of the thigh forwards. Do not flex at the hip.

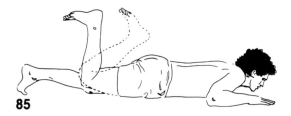

85

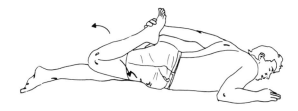

85. **Quadriceps stretch and hip mobility: lying.** Try to keep the back as flat as possible while you let the heel come back towards the buttocks. If you arch, stop and repeat the exercise without arching. Progress by clasping onto the foot, repeat with the other hand. Make sure the heel comes back towards the buttocks on this side, not to the opposite side. Continue this stretch by letting the leg fall in then outwards when the knee is at 90 degrees. This improves hip flexibility. Do not let the buttocks lift or pelvis roll as the leg drops inwards or outwards. Each leg should have the same amount of rotation. Now repeat the quadriceps stretch.

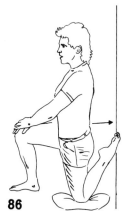

86

86. **Hip flexor stretch: kneeling** — for quadriceps and iliopsoas; can be done with or without a wall. Use the hand if there is no wall. Kneeling with one foot behind, top of the foot against the wall, flatten the back and shift the top of the thigh forward. Posteriorly tilt the pelvis, that is, pull the abdomen up and inwards. An excellent exercise if you get anterior groin or hip pain.

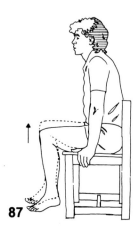

87

87. Hip flexor (iliopsoas) strengthening. While sitting, try to lift one knee to the roof. Try to maintain a slightly lordotic curve as you do this. This exercise is useful if you have a sway back posture, where the iliopsoas is very overstretched and weak. Sometimes it needs to be used for flat back posture too.

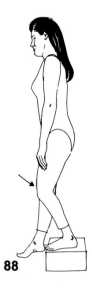

88

88. Step strengthening exercise. Stand on a step and tighten the quadriceps as you bend and straighten the knee. Particularly try to tighten the inside muscle (vastus medialis) as usually this is weakest. Use the other leg as a lever by extending it down over the step. Strengthening of this muscle, combined with stretching the hip abductors (exercise 61) and strengthening the lateral rotators of the hip (exercise 64), can assist if you suffer from 'runner's knee' (pain under the knee-cap).

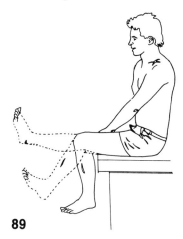

89

89. **Inner range quadriceps strengthening.** While sitting, place your hand on the inside of the quadriceps (vastus medialis) and let the leg drop down 25–30 degrees. Contract this muscle and use it to raise the leg to horizontal again. Have the foot turned out slightly as you lock and straighten the knee. Flex the foot.

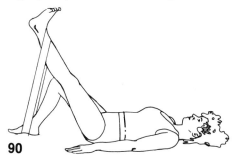

90

90. **Quadriceps strengthening.** Lying, pull the toes back. Tighten the quadriceps and lift the leg. Repeat but do not let the leg touch the ground when it is lowered. A rubber band or weight on the foot will make this exercise more effective. Bend the knee of the lower leg if a band is used, OR on the elbows or hands, tighten the quadriceps and do leg lifts. Do not let the knee bend on the out-stretched leg.

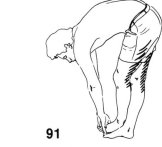

91

91. **Hamstring stretch.** Standing, let the knees bend as you touch your toes. Now straighten one then the other. Do not bounce. Now cross the legs and repeat to stretch both hamstrings.

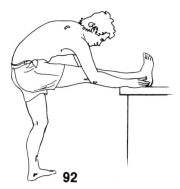

92. **Alternative hamstring stretch.** Standing, rest the leg on a chair or table, and gently lean forward, keeping the back straight. Bend the other knee to increase the stretch. Do not bend forward from the upper back only. Not recommended if you have a thoracic kyphosis.

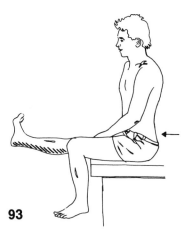

93. **Hamstring stretch: sitting.** While sitting, curve the lower back inwards and straighten one leg. Try to pull the toes back to stretch tight calf muscles. Excellent exercise to stretch the hamstrings if you have a thoracic kyphosis or a flat back posture.

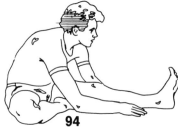

94. **Hamstring and lower back stretch.** With one foot on the inside of the thigh of the outstretched leg, place hands on either side of it. Gently try to bend the elbows and ease forward. Do not just curve the head and shoulders forward.

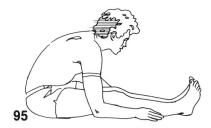

95. **Advanced hamstring and lower back stretch.** Progress to both legs straight and with flat back, ease forward, aiming to bend the elbows. Always keep the hands resting on the feet or beside the legs to support the back as you lean forward.

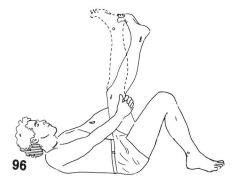

96. **Single leg hamstring stretch.** Raise one leg up, clasp behind the knee, just below it. Now try to straighten the leg, pulling the ankle back towards you. Not recommended if you have flat back posture. Once you can stretch the leg to 90 degrees, straighten the other leg. You may use a towel around the foot to assist with this stretch.

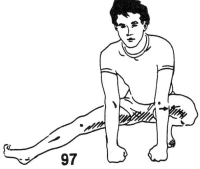

97. **Combined hamstring and adductor stretch.** This stretches both adductors and hamstrings. Come up on the toes of one leg, bend the knee and bring the buttocks towards the floor on this side. Pull the toes back on the outstretched leg and keep the elbow inside the bent leg to provide counter-resistance.

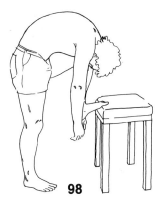

98. Upper hamstring stretch. Standing, bend one leg up onto a chair, then let the head and shoulders drop forwards onto the inside of the thigh. Drop the ankle to the floor, just resting the toes on the chair to increase the stretch. The weight-bearing knee can be bent if you cannot feel an effective stretch with it straight.

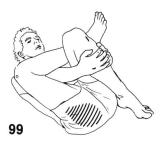

99. Upper hamstring stretch: lying. Cross one ankle in front of a bent knee. Now put both hands through and around the bent leg and hug this knee up onto the chest. Counter-resist the ankle against the knee to increase the effectiveness of the stretch. You should feel it at the top of the hamstring and the base of the buttocks.

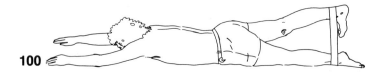

100. Hamstring strengthening. Lying prone, raise one leg behind. Be sure not to arch the back so that gluteus maximus does all the work. Use a weight or rubber band to be more effective.

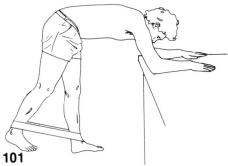

101.

101. **Standing hamstring strengthening with resistance.** Bend at the waist and rest the elbows on a table. With a band around the ankles pull one leg behind.

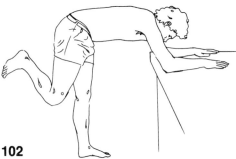

102

102. **Hamstring curl with resistance.** Repeat exercise 101 with the leg bent.

 Calves

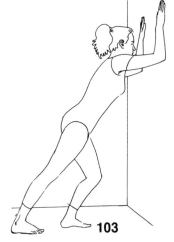

103

103. **Calf stretch** — gastrocnemius. Leaning against a wall, lift the arch of the foot slightly. Keep the hip and the knee in a straight line and lean forward. Stretch each leg separately. Do not let the arch collapse to a flat footed position as you do this stretch, as this may cause overstretched ligaments in the foot, leading to an overpronated foot. This should be avoided.

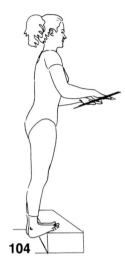

104

104. **Step stretch.** Standing on the edge of a step, slowly lower the heels over the edge of the step. Repeat with foot turned out, then inwards slightly to stretch both heads of gastrocnemius.

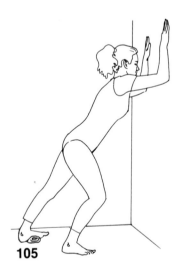

105

105. **Combined gastrocnemius/peroneal stretch.** Place a small object such as a crepe bandage under the arch of the foot. Keep the heel on the floor. Now lean forward keeping the knee straight. Hold for 6–10 seconds, then bend the knee. If you get sore calves or achilles tendon after sport this exercise is ideal for you.

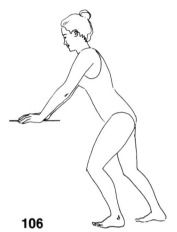

106

106. **Achilles and soleus stretch.** Same position as exercise 103, now bend the knee to stretch the achilles tendon and soleus.

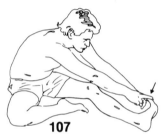

107

107. **Deep toe flexor stretch** — flexor hallicus longus. While sitting, place the hand under the first toe and stretch it back towards the ankle. Stiffness at the base of the big toe (it should bend back 60–90 degrees) can cause pain in the arch (called plantafascitis) or 'shin splints'.

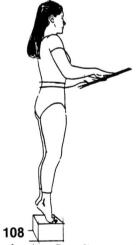

108

108. **Toe raises** — calf strengthening. Standing, use the calf muscle as you raise up and down. Do not let the arch of the foot collapse inwards throughout the exercise.

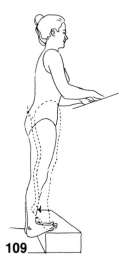

109

109. **Calf stretch and strengthening.** On a step, let the ankle drop below the step level. (Feel the stretch on the calf.) Repeat the toe raise. Repeat with single leg as well as both legs.

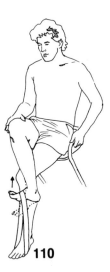

110

110. **Shin strengthening with a resistance** — tibialis anterior, extensor digitorium and extensor hallicus longus. Using a low stool or a box, tuck one foot under a band wrapped around the box. Now use the front muscles of the shin to lift the band. Use the other leg to keep the band down. The same exercise can be done without a box and just using the band and crossing the legs can make the exercise harder.

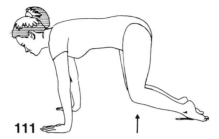

111

111. **Shin strengthening.** Kneeling with palms on the floor, use the top of the foot and anterior shin muscles to lift the body weight.

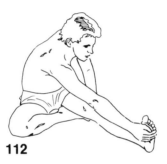

112

112. **Peroneals stretch.** While sitting, one leg bent, use the hand opposite the outstretched leg placed on the outside of the foot, to pull the toes and ankle inwards. Keep the ankle flexed at 90 degrees.

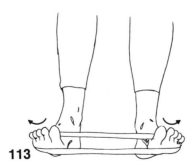

113

113. **Peroneals strengthening.** Place an elastic band around the forefoot and pull the toes up and outwards. Keep the legs apart to be effective. An excellent exercise, combined with exercises 114 and 115 if you have weak ankles which you sprain or injure often.

Feet

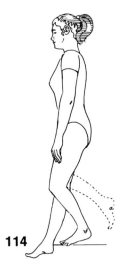

114

114. Ankle strengthening and balance. While standing, bend one leg. Go up on the toe and try to bend the knee directly over the foot. Do not let the arch of the foot collapse. You may need to hold on to something for balance, but only initially. To increase the difficulty of the exercise, close your eyes as you do it, or bounce a ball against a wall or on the ground, while you are up on your toe.

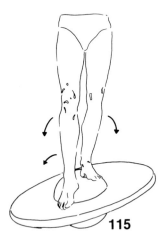

115

115. Wobble board — balance and proprioception. Use both feet initially, then progress to one foot and work the ankle in all directions. Try to hold on to something only minimally and if possible not at all. Using a few pillows on top of each other is ideal if you do not have access to a wobble board. When this feels too easy, try to do this with your eyes closed. Be careful though!

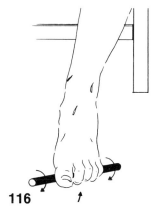

116

116. **Intrinsic foot strengthening.** While sitting, try to pick up pens or a towel to strengthen the intrinsic muscles of the foot. An ideal exercise if you have flat feet, as it strengthens the muscles which support the arch of the foot.

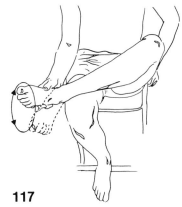

117

117. **Ankle mobility.** Clasp onto one foot and loosen the ankle and foot by rotating it in circles one way, then the other, then loosen the bones in the fore-foot with your hand by flexing and extending them. An ideal exercise if your feet are tired at the end of a working day.

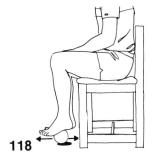

118

118. **Stretching the arch of the foot.** While sitting, place a golf or tennis ball under the arch of the foot, then roll it forwards and back, controlling it with the toes.

EXERCISES NOT RECOMMENDED
AND SAFE ALTERNATIVES

Any exercise performed at high speed with lack of control can create instability around a joint and musculoskeletal problems may develop. Always work at a controlled pace with good form when you are exercising. Consult a sports specialist if you are getting pain with a particular exercise. It may be inappropriate for your body type. An exercise may cause discomfort but it should not cause pain!

The following exercises are not recommended as they can be potentially harmful, particularly when performed at high speed or with high repetitions. Safe alternatives are suggested.

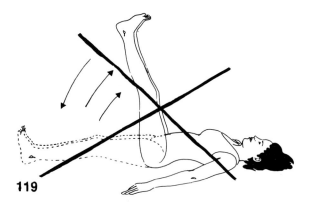

119. **Double straight leg raise** — incorrect. Double straight leg raises with back arched are stressful for the lower back, because iliopsoas is worked in a shortened range if sufficient strength in the abdominals is not present.

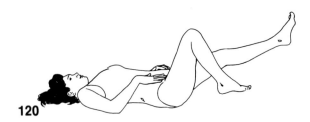

120. **Inner range leg cycling** — correct. As an alternative to exercise 119, work only in the range where you can maintain a flat back. Working between 45 and 90 degrees from the floor is acceptable if the back can be maintained flat on the floor. Bracing the abdominals will prevent arching of the back.

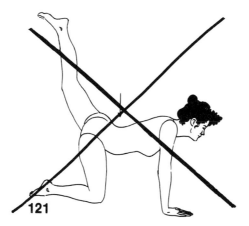

121. **Hip hyperextension** — incorrect. Hip hyperextension often performed in aerobics classes at high speed, with no control, is potentially stressful to the lower back — ligaments, muscles and the discs.

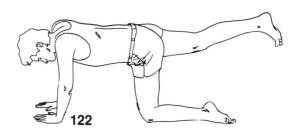

122. **Gluteus maximus strengthening** — correct. (Alternative to exercise 121.) Control the movement by flexing the foot and resting down on the elbows, keeping the buttocks tight also reduces stress on the back. Do not move greater than 10 degrees beyond the vertical. Using a bent leg to perform this exercise can also be used as an alternative to strengthening the gluteus maximus. Do not let the foot twist in or out as this can stress the lower back or hip joint area, and do not hyperextend the lumbar spine.

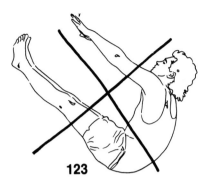

123

123. **Straight leg and jack-knife sit-ups** — incorrect. Performed at high speed with high repetitions, these exercises can be potentially stressful on the lower back because it tightens and strengthens iliopsoas and does not permit the abdominals and the rectus femoris muscle to work through their full range. A lordotic curve in the lower back may result if the iliopsoas is tight. While jack-knife sit-ups should never be done, straight leg sit-ups are permissible if performed in a controlled manner, not at speed. They should never be used in fitness classes where the control of speed is not possible.

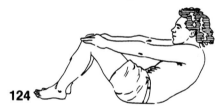

124

124. **Bent-leg sit-ups** — correct. These sit-ups are a safe alternative to the sit-ups in exercise 123. Exercises 69–79 show how to isolate and strengthen both the upper and lower segments of the abdominals, effectively and safely.

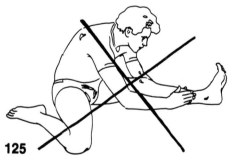

125

125. **Hurdler's stretch** — incorrect. This is where one leg is outstretched and the other leg is bent at the knee and turned backwards. There is potential damage to the medial structures of the knee, in this position. To stretch the hamstrings and lower back, always turn the knee outwards with the foot resting on the inside of the outstretched leg.

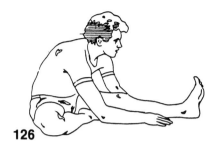

126. **Hamstring stretch** — correct. With one foot on the inside of the thigh of the outstretched leg, place hands on either side of it. Gently try to bend the elbows and ease forward. Do not just curve the head and shoulders forward. Keep the back straight.

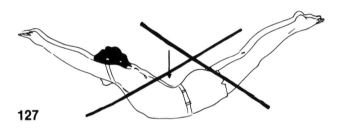

127. **Back hyperextension** — incorrect. Raising the legs and arms at the same time places unnecessary stress on the lower back. Working the arms then the legs, either independently or opposites, is less stressful.

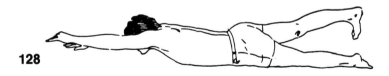

128. **Opposite arm and leg** — correct. Stretch them out long, rather than arching too far. Repeat both sides.

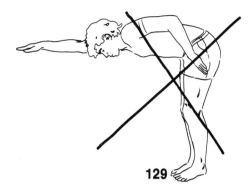

129. **Sustained forward flexion** — bouncing while touching the toes — incorrect. Sustained forward flexion is a position often used in fitness classes. However, it overloads the discs in the lumbar spine. It should only be used as a stretch if at all, not as a position for working the arms. Touching the toes and bouncing to get further should never be attempted.

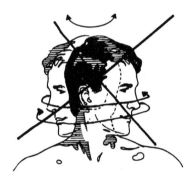

130. **Circular neck rotations** — incorrect. Rotating the neck through a full circle one way then the other, can close down some of the joints in the cervical spine and impinge on the nerve structures. Exercises 1, 2 and 3 show how to exercise the cervical spine correctly and safely.

6 — DAILY ROUTINES

This chapter shows the exercises suitable for daily muscle maintenance. If you have not exercised for some time, start with level 1. When you find these too easy, progress to level 2, then to level 3. If you currently exercise regularly, practise level 1, but you should be able to move to either level 2 or 3 quite quickly. The number of repetitions is written in parentheses for every exercise.

Sometimes it is not possible to play sport every day, so following these regimes can ensure you are keeping your muscles fit daily.

Try to spend 10–15 minutes morning and evening on these daily routines:

Minimum — three times per week, once per day.

Maximum — twice daily, 15–20 minutes.

LEVEL 1 — BEGINNERS

Warm-up

Circle your arms forwards and backwards eight to ten times. Repeat. While standing, hug one knee up to your chest, then the other. Use a stationary bicycle or mini-trampoline to work out on for 10–12 minutes. Going for a brisk walk will also prepare you for the following exercises.

Mobility exercises and stretches

1. Neck flexion (×1)
2. Neck extension (×1)
3. Neck rotation (×1)
4. Neck side flexion (×1)
17. Thoracic spine and shoulder mobility exercise (×3–4)
21. Tricep stretch (×3–4)
22. Latissimus dorsi stretch (×3–4)
23. Shoulder rotations: sitting (×4–5)
25. Shoulder shrugs (×2–3)
84. Quadriceps stretch (hold for 6–10 secs)
93. Hamstring stretch: sitting (×2–3)
49. Knee hug stretch (×4–5)
46. Lower back release (×4–5)

48. Pelvis and lower back release (×4–5)
50. Spinal rotation stretch: lying (hold for 6–10 secs each side)
36. Cat stretch: extension (×2–3)
37. Cat stretch: flexion (×2–3)
38. Lower back release (×1)

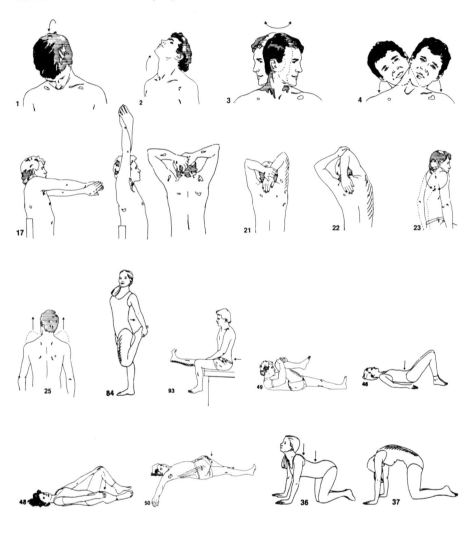

Strengthening exercises

55. Opposite arm and leg lift ($\times 4-6$)
69. Sit-ups ($\times 4-6$)
73. Beginners' lower abdominals strengthening ($\times 4-5$)
78. Adductor stretch and oblique strengthening ($\times 4-5$)
63. Hip strengthening ($\times 4-5$)
 6. Wall exercise ($\times 4-6$)
117. Ankle mobility

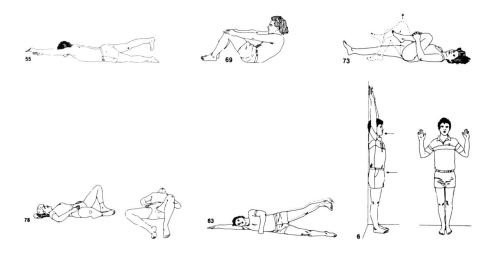

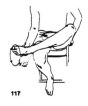

LEVEL 2 — INTERMEDIATE

Warm-up

Loosen up the arms with large circular movements. Try incorporating a light jog, a brisk walk, skipping or cycling prior to trying the following exercises. Include these exercises into your daily regime if you are already currently engaged in a fitness programme.

Mobility exercises and stretches

1. Neck flexion ($\times 1$)
2. Neck extension ($\times 1$)
3. Neck rotation ($\times 1$)
4. Neck side flexion ($\times 1$)
5. Neck stretch ($\times 2$)
17. Thoracic spine and shoulder mobility exercise ($\times 3-4$)
21. Tricep stretch ($\times 3-4$)
22. Latissimus dorsi stretch ($\times 3-4$)
23. Shoulder rotations: sitting ($\times 2-3$)
25. Shoulder shrugs ($\times 2-3$)
93. Hamstring stretch: sitting (hold for 6–10 secs, $\times 2-3$)
36. Cat stretch: extension ($\times 2-3$)
    (not recommended if you have back pain)
37. Cat stretch: flexion ($\times 2-3$)
    (not recommended if you have back pain)
11. Pectoral stretch (hold for 6–10 secs, $\times 2-3$)
40. Passive back extension stretch ($\times 4-5$)
19. Shoulder and scapula mobility ($\times 3-4$)
20. Shoulder and thoracic spine mobility ($\times 2-3$)
50. Spinal rotation stretch: lying (hold for 6–10 secs each side, $\times 2-3$)
99. Upper hamstring stretch: lying ($\times 2-3$)
38. Lower back release (hold for 20 secs, $\times 1$)

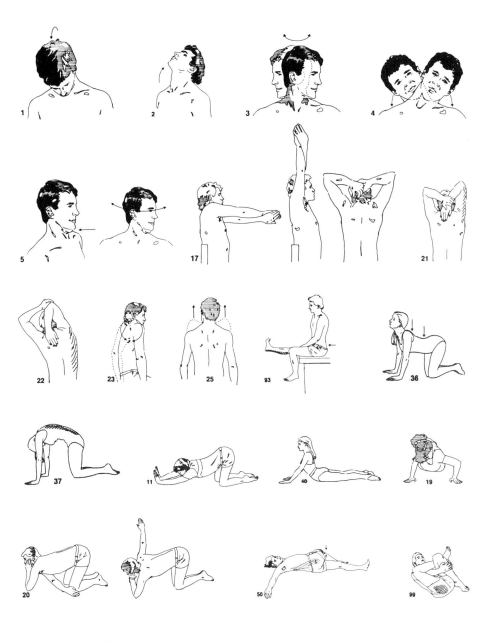

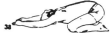

Strengthening exercises

   6. Wall exercise (×6–8)
69. Sit-ups (×8–10)
74. Intermediate lower abdominals strengthening (×8–10)
78. Adductor stretch and oblique strengthening (×8–10)
63. Hip strengthening (×8–10)
12. Pectoral and tricep strengthening (×8–10)
13. Shoulder girdle strengthening (×6–8)

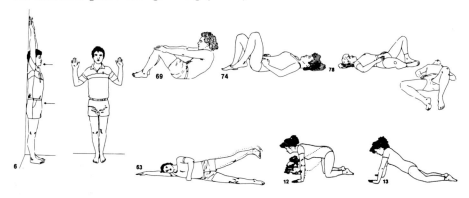

LEVEL 3 — ADVANCED

Warm-up

Jogging, brisk walking, cycling or skipping for 15–30 minutes prior to trying the following exercises is recommended. The exercises in this section are only suitable if you have completed levels 1 and 2 easily, and if you are currently on a fitness programme.

Mobility exercises and stretches

   1. Neck flexion (×1)
   2. Neck extension (×1)
   3. Neck rotation (×1)
   4. Neck side flexion (×1)
   5. Neck stretch (×1)

17. Thoracic spine and shoulder mobility exercise (×2)
21. Tricep stretch (×2–3)
22. Latissimus dorsi stretch (×2–3)
23. Shoulder rotations: sitting (×2–3)
25. Shoulder shrugs (×2–3)
34. Advanced thoracic spine mobility (×2–3)
32. Latissimus dorsi/quadratus lumborum stretch (×4–6)
7. Neck extensor and upper back strengthening (×4–6)
36. Cat stretch: extension (×2–3)
37. Cat stretch: flexion (×2–3)
59. Hip stretch for piriformis and sciatica (×2–3)
39. Spinal flexion/extension stretch (×1)
19. Shoulder and scapula mobility (×2)
44. Spinal stretch and abdominal strengthening: bent legs (×2)
99. Upper hamstring stretch: lying (×2–3)
60. Advanced hip stretch (×2–3)
38. Lower back release (hold for 15 secs, ×1)
80. Adductor stretch: standing/squatting (×2–3)

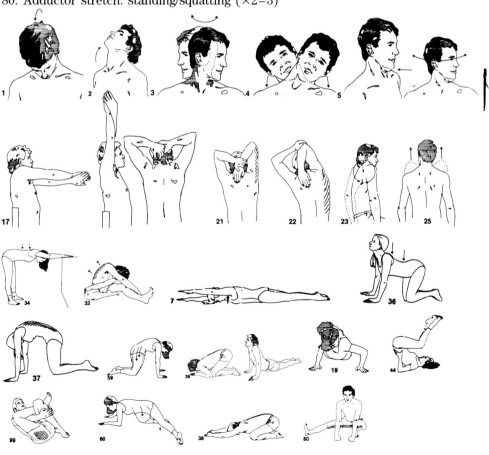

Strengthening exercises

  6. Wall exercise (×8–10)
12. Pectoral and tricep strengthening (×8–10)
13. Shoulder girdle strengthening (×8–10)
14. Full push-up (×12–5, progress to two sets)
55. Opposite arm and leg lift (×8–10)
65. Buttocks strengthening (×6–8)
63. Hip strengthening (×6–8)
69. Sit-ups (×12–15)
73. Beginners' lower abdominals strengthening (×6–8) *OR*
74. Intermediate lower abdominals strengthening (×6–8)
75. Advanced lower abdominals strengthening (×8–10)
77. Combination oblique strengthening (×8–10 each side)
38. Lower back release (hold for 20 secs, ×1)

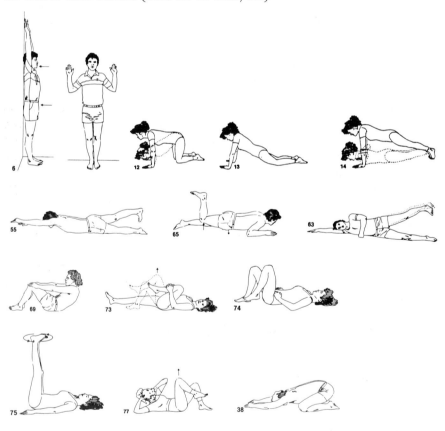

7 — EXERCISES FOR SPECIAL GROUPS

This chapter will provide exercises for special groups, including postural types, hypermobile (overflexible) people, over-50s, the traveller and desk worker, musicians, children and also for healthy back care.

The exercises are shown in the order of sequence in which you are to perform them. The number of repetitions is included in parentheses for each exercise.

THE TRAVELLER AND DESK WORKER

Within the confined space of the plane, train or car, or working at a desk all day, when you are restricted to just sitting for extended periods of time, the body can become very stiff in its muscles and joints. The exercises shown below can minimise this effect. Try to practise them whenever possible, either during your trip or as a break from your desk work.

Try to keep the body moving as much as possible within the confined space. In the plane or train, go for regular walks. In the car, take a rest break every 2–3 hours at a minimum, and stretch the body and go for a walk. Use a back support or a small towel rolled up and placed in the small of your back to support your back when sitting.

Take breaks from your desk at a minimum of every half an hour for 5–8 minutes, especially if you are working on a computer or typing. Go for a walk in your breaks.

Exercises for the traveller and desk worker

1. Neck flexion (×1)
2. Neck extension (×1)
3. Neck rotation (×1)
5. Neck stretch (×2)
21. Tricep stretch (×2–3)
22. Latissimus dorsi stretch (×2–3)
23. Shoulder rotations: sitting (×2–3)
25. Shoulder shrugs (×2–3)

119

26. Wrist, shoulder and neck stretch (hold for 6–10 secs, ×2–3)
    When driving or travelling in a plane, take a break and try some of these
    exercises.
34. Advanced thoracic spine mobility (×2–3)
93. Hamstring stretch: sitting (hold for 6–10 secs, ×2–3)
103. Calf stretch (hold for 6–10 secs, ×2–3)
117. Ankle mobility (×3–4)
15. Isometric pectoral strengthening (×2–3)
16. Pectoral and shoulder strengthening: sitting (×2–3)

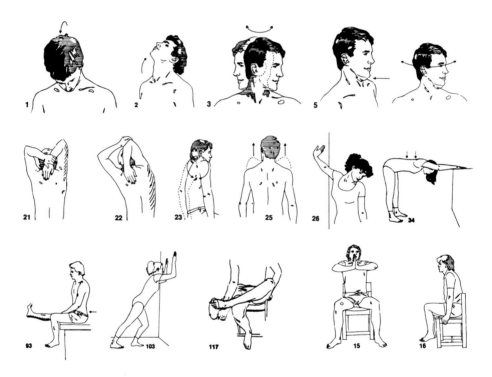

HEALTHY BACK CARE

Warm-up

Perform some large circular movements of the arms, 9–10 forward and then back. Bend the knees 5–10 degrees to take the load off the back while you are exercising the arms. With hands on knees, circle one way and then the other. Take deep breaths in and stretch the arms and hands above the head. Exhale as you let the arms come down by the side to relax.

Only try aerobic activity advised by a health professional. Swimming is usually the ideal for a painful back but do not sustain one stroke for a long period of time as this can place too much load on the back. Try to vary the strokes you do. Do not try any stroke which aggravates your back. These exercises are designed to be preventative and are not a cure for your backache. You should consult a health practitioner if you suffer from backache.

Stretch your calves, hamstrings, hip flexors and lower back.

Strengthen upper and lower abdominals and back extensors of both the neck and lower back.

Check your posture (see Chapter 3 to identify your postural type) and perform the exercises in this chapter for your type.

Repeat the wall exercise (exercise 6) to check your posture daily.

Check your home and work environment: the height of chairs, desks etc.

Have a massage regularly.

Exercise regularly — include aerobic exercise in your programme.

Try not to sit for prolonged periods. Take regular breaks if your job is sedentary. Try the exercises recommended for travellers and desk workers in this chapter.

If pain persists, see a specialist.

Find ways to manage your own back complaint. If you know what the problem is, establish what helps your back, which exercises make it feel better and which ones aggravate the problem. Do not keep trying to find a label or answer for your discomfort from different health professionals. Start exercising within your pain limit and see if this reduces your pain.

Exercises for healthy back care

Stretches

36. Cat stretch: extension (×2–3)
37. Cat stretch: flexion (×2–3)
48. Pelvis and lower back release
49. Knee hug stretch
51. Double leg spinal rotation (×3–4 each side)
50. Spinal rotation stretch: lying (hold for 6–10 secs, ×2–3)
59. Hip stretch for piriformis and sciatica (×2–3)

93. Hamstring stretch: sitting (hold for 6–10 secs, ×2–3)
99. Upper hamstring stretch: lying (×2–3)
40. Passive back extension stretch (×5–8)
38. Lower back release (hold for 10–15 secs)
32. Latissimus dorsi/quadratus lumborum stretch (×2–3) OR
33. Side trunk stretch (×2–3)

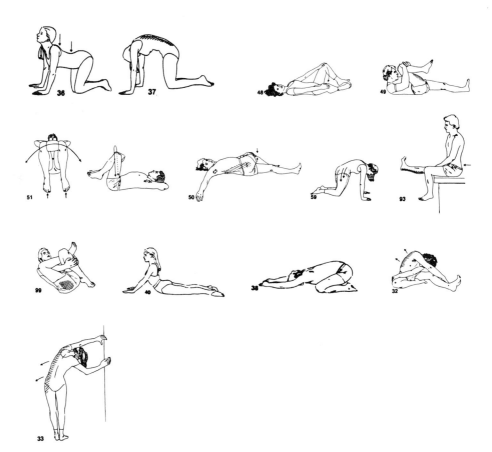

Strengthening exercises

53. Back strengthening single leg lift (×4–5)
54. Back strengthening single arm lift (×4–5)
55. Opposite arm and leg lift (×6–8)
64. Lateral rotators strengthening of the hip (×6–8)
69. Sit-ups (×8–10)
73. Beginners' lower abdominals strengthening (×6–8)
74. Intermediate lower abdominals strengthening (×6–8)
78. Adductor stretch and oblique strengthening (×6–8)
 6. Wall exercise (×4–5)

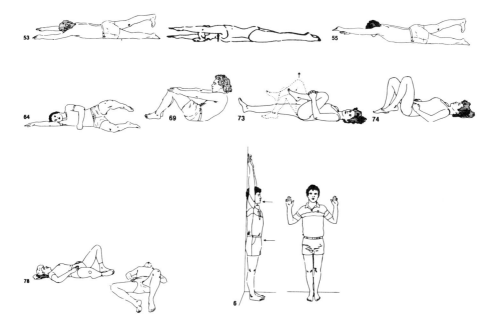

MUSICIANS

Playing a musical instrument, whether it be guitar, piano, the flute or any other instrument, usually requires many hours sitting in a fixed position. Even if you are a conductor you will benefit from these exercises.

Try to take breaks whenever possible when you are practising and practise the following exercises. Spend a little more time on the stretches which affect the areas and muscles where you currently feel stiffness when you are playing or practising.

Exercises for musicians

Stretches

    1. Neck flexion ($\times 2-3$)
    2. Neck extension ($\times 2-3$)
    3. Neck rotation ($\times 2-3$)
    4. Neck side flexion ($\times 2-3$)
    5. Neck stretch ($\times 2$)
  17. Thoracic spine and shoulder mobility exercise ($\times 4$)
  21. Tricep stretch ($\times 2-3$)
  22. Latissimus dorsi stretch ($\times 2-3$)
  23. Shoulder rotations: sitting ($\times 2-3$)
  25. Shoulder shrugs ($\times 2-3$)
  28. Thoracic spine and rhomboids stretch ($\times 4-6$)
  26. Wrist, shoulder and neck stretch (hold for 6–10 secs, $\times 3-4$)
  27. Wrist and finger stretch ($\times 6-8$)
  33. Side trunk stretch ($\times 2-3$)
  18. Thoracic spine and shoulder mobility using a rod ($\times 3-4$)
  34. Advanced thoracic spine mobility ($\times 2-3$)
  93. Hamstring stretch: sitting (hold for 6–10 secs, $\times 2-3$)
      Can be performed during practice sessions.
117. Ankle mobility ($\times 3-4$)
  36. Cat stretch: extension ($\times 3-4$)
  37. Cat stretch: flexion ($\times 3-4$)
  40. Passive back extension stretch ($\times 6-8$)
  49. Knee hug stretch ($\times 4-6$)
  50. Spinal rotation stretch: lying (hold for 6–10 secs, $\times 2-3$)
  29. Upper back stretch (hold for 6–10 secs, $\times 2-3$)

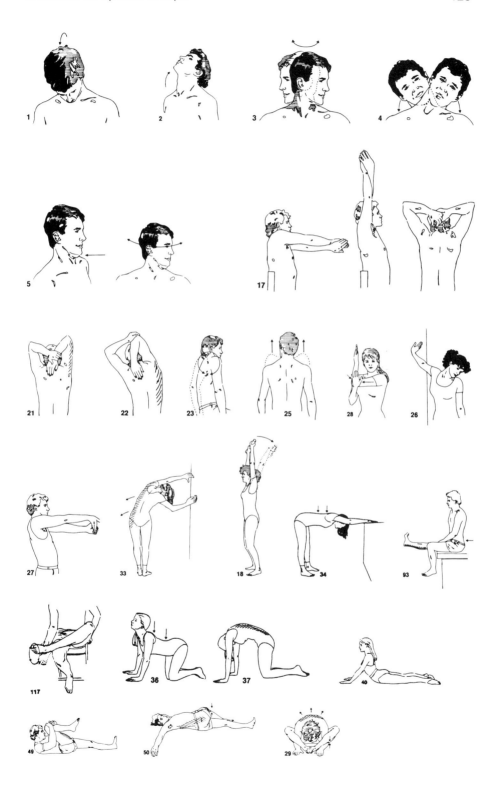

Strengthening exercises

15. Isometric pectoral strengthening ($\times3-4$)
13. Shoulder girdle strengthening ($\times4-6$)
53. Back strengthening single leg lift ($\times3-4$)
54. Back strengthening single arm lift ($\times6-8$)
55. Opposite arm and leg lift ($\times8-10$)
74. Intermediate lower abdominals strengthening ($\times4-6$)
79. Advanced adductor stretch and oblique strengthening ($\times6-8$)
33. Side trunk stretch (hold for $6-10$ secs, $\times2-3$)

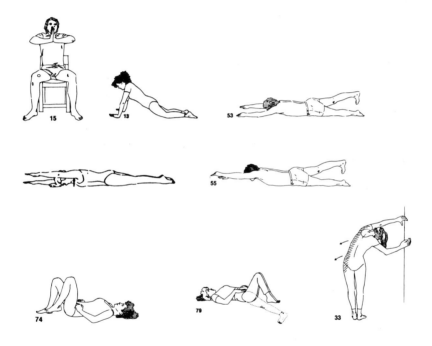

THE OVER-50s

Warm-up

Go for a 15–20 minute walk or bicycle ride, or just circle the arms, both forwards and backwards, 8–10 times each way. Then try to hug each knee onto the chest (while standing, if possible). Bend the knees slightly and rotate them each way. Loosen the ankles and feet by rotating them with your hands while you are sitting. Be gentle on your body when you try these exercises. No exercise should cause pain. Try to do these exercises at least once a day.

Work within your own limits. Be gentle, and do not bounce. Take all the stretches through the full range.

Push to discomfort but not through pain. If you are uncertain if any of the exercises are harmful to you, check with a health professional.

Perform all the exercises on a carpeted floor, not a soft bed.

If you have arthritis, be gentle in your exercising and try to become involved in an aquarobics class, swimming or brisk walking to maintain cardiovascular fitness and to keep your muscles supple and strong. Pain from arthritis can be markedly reduced if you keep fit. Arthritis itself is usually the result of inactivity, and far less often from excessive activity. Exercising regularly will improve circulation through the body and keeping flexible and strong will reduce the stress taken by the affected joints.

Exercises for the over-50s

Stretches

  1. Neck flexion ($\times 1$)
  2. Neck extension ($\times 1$)
  3. Neck rotation ($\times 1$)
  4. Neck side flexion ($\times 1$)
  5. Neck stretch ($\times 2$)
21. Tricep stretch ($\times 2$–3)
22. Latissimus dorsi stretch ($\times 2$–3)
23. Shoulder rotations: sitting ($\times 2$–3) *OR*
24. Shoulder rotations: lying ($\times 2$–3)
28. Thoracic spine and rhomboids stretch ($\times 2$–3)
25. Shoulder shrugs ($\times 2$–3)
26. Wrist, shoulder and neck stretch ($\times 2$–3)
85. Quadricep stretch and hip mobility: lying ($\times 4$–5 each leg)
93. Hamstring stretch: sitting (hold for 6–10 secs, $\times 2$–3)
36. Cat stretch: extension ($\times 2$–3)
37. Cat stretch: flexion ($\times 2$–3)
38. Lower back release ($\times 2$–3)
40. Passive back extension stretch ($\times 4$–5)

49. Knee hug stretch (×4–5)
51. Double leg spinal rotation (×3–4 each side)
78. Adductor stretch and oblique strengthening (×3–4)
48. Pelvis and lower back release (×4–5)

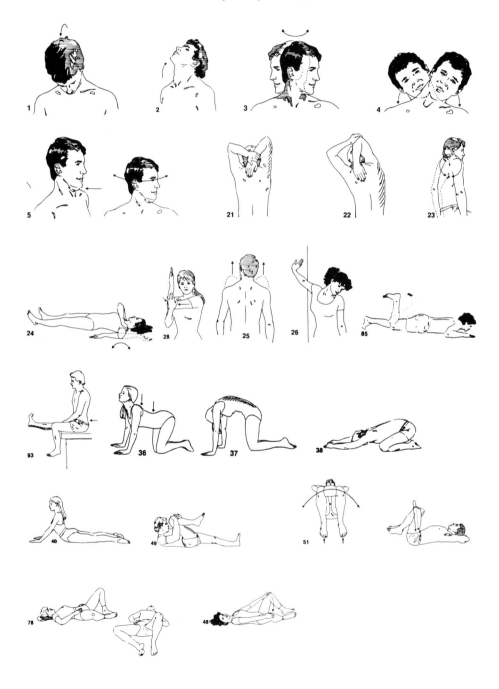

Strengthening exercises

  6. Wall exercise (×3–4)

12. Pectoral and tricep strengthening (×2–3)

53. Back strengthening single leg lift (×4–5)

54. Back strengthening single arm lift (×4–5)

55. Opposite arm and leg lift (×4–6)

64. Lateral rotators strengthening (×4–5)

63. Hip strengthening (×4–5)

73. Beginners' lower abdominals strengthening

Finish your exercise routine with exercise 38 — lower back release.

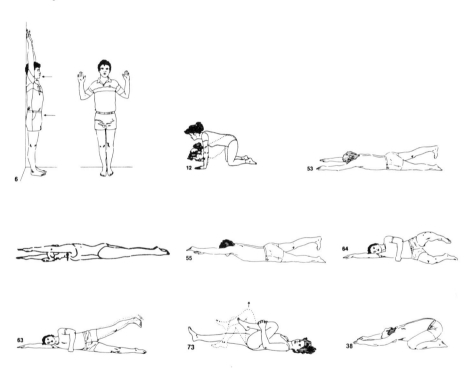

CHILDREN

In the teenage years it is important to stretch muscles prior to whatever sport you play. Before adolescence, children should not need overemphasis on stretching, provided they participate regularly in some form of aerobic, fun sport. This should be sufficient for them to retain their flexibility.

Focus in the younger years (under 12) should be on agility and co-ordination skills. The ideal for any child is to participate in a variety of sports and activities. Using a trampoline is an ideal way to develop balance, control and co-ordination and strength around the joints.

The following exercises are more suited to those older than 9–10 years. It is highly recommended that children practise some form of exercise daily — 10–15 minutes is sufficient and could be incorporated into a child's daily school programme.

Remember, it is important that no exercise should hurt.

Children's exercises

Stretches

1. Neck flexion ($\times 1$)
2. Neck extension ($\times 1$)
3. Neck rotation ($\times 1$)
4. Neck side flexion ($\times 1$)
6. Wall exercise ($\times 6-8$ daily) This exercise is excellent for reviewing children's posture as they are growing.
17. Thoracic spine and shoulder mobility exercise ($\times 2-3$)
21. Tricep stretch ($\times 2-3$)
22. Latissimus dorsi stretch ($\times 2-3$)
23. Shoulder rotations: sitting ($\times 2-3$)
25. Shoulder shrugs ($\times 2-3$)
93. Hamstring stretch: sitting (hold for 6–10 secs, $\times 2-3$)
29. Upper back stretch ($\times 2$)
84. Quadriceps stretch ($\times 2-3$ each leg, hold for 6–10 secs)
36. Cat stretch: extension ($\times 2-3$)
37. Cat stretch: flexion ($\times 2-3$)
39. Spinal flexion/extension stretch ($\times 1$)
38. Lower back release (hold for 10–12 secs, $\times 1$)
41. Lower back stretch ($\times 2-3$)
51. Double leg spinal rotation ($\times 2-3$ each side)
50. Spinal rotation stretch: lying (hold for 6–10 secs each side, $\times 1$)
49. Knee hug stretch ($\times 3$ each leg)
80. Adductor stretch: standing/squatting ($\times 2$)
81. Adductor stretch: sitting ($\times 2$)

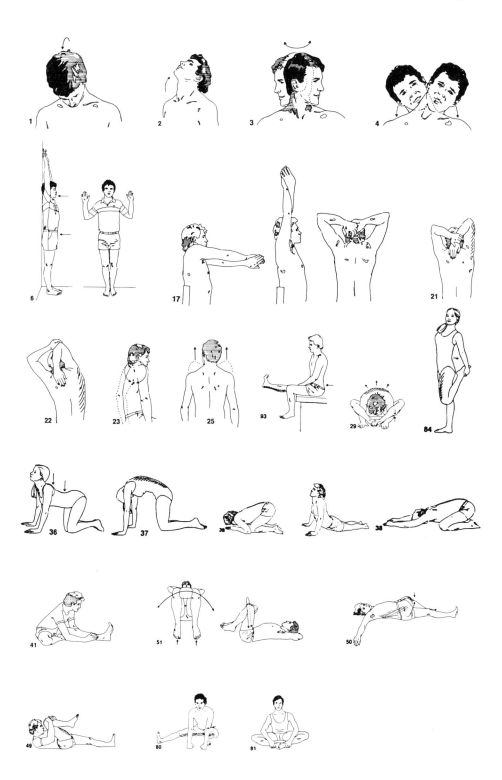

Strengthening exercises

73. Beginners' lower abdominals strengthening ($\times 4-5$)
78. Adductor strength and oblique strengthening ($\times 4-5$)
55. Opposite arm and leg lift strengthening ($\times 4-5$)

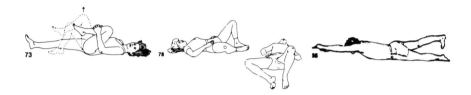

HYPERMOBILITY

These exercises are *only* for those who are hypermobile (that is, very flexible in all your joints). If you can sit with your legs outstretched and can bend forward so your head can rest on your knees, then these exercises are suitable for you. Consult a health professional if you are unsure. (See Chapter 2 for details about hypermobility).

If you are hypermobile but not used to exercising, start with level 1. If you are currently involved in a fitness programme you should still start with level 1 but can move to level 2 if you find the first level too easy.

The exercises will help prevent problems occurring at your unstable, over-flexible joints. Even though you are flexible you need to work your muscles through their full range to balance your flexibility with strength. When stretching, do so with control at the end of the range. Do not force your muscles past their end range or you may overstretch the ligaments supporting the joint.

Warm-up

Large circular movements with the arms, going for a brisk walk or using a bicycle are helpful warm-up activities.

Level 1 — exercises for hypermobility

Strengthening exercises

73. Beginners' lower abdominals strengthening ($\times 6-8$)
74. Intermediate lower abdominals strengthening ($\times 8-10$)
77. Combination oblique strengthening ($\times 8-10$)
78. Adductor stretch and oblique strengthening ($\times 2-3$)
68. Alternate cycling exercise ($\times 8-10$)
63. Hip strengthening ($\times 8-10$)
64. Lateral rotators of the hip ($\times 8-10$)
65. Buttock strengthening ($\times 6-8$)
53. Back strengthening single leg lift ($\times 6$)
54. Back strengthening single arm lift ($\times 4-6$)
55. Opposite arm and leg lift strengthening ($\times 6-8$)
56. Alternate swimming back strengthening ($\times 6-8$)

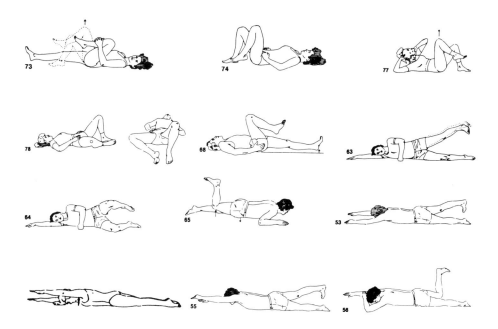

Stretches

97. Combined hamstring and adductor stretch (×2 each side)
93. Hamstring stretch: sitting (hold for 6–10 secs, ×2–3)
32. Latissimus dorsi/quadratus lumborum stretch (×2–3)
50. Spinal rotation stretch: lying (×2–3)
34. Advanced thoracic spine mobility (×2)
49. Knee hug stretch (×6–8 each leg)
48. Pelvis and lower back release (×2)
38. Lower back release (hold for 10–15 secs, ×1)
 6. Wall exercise (×6–8)

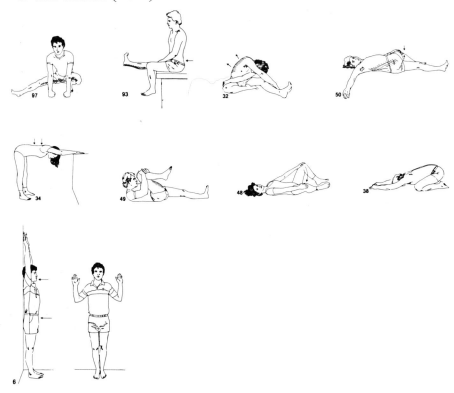

Level 2 — exercises for hypermobility

Strengthening exercises

44. Spinal stretch and abdominals strengthening: bent legs (×3–4)
45. Advanced spinal stretch and abdominals strengthening: straight legs (×3–4)
74. Intermediate lower abdominals strengthening (×4–6)
75. Advanced lower abdominals strengthening (×8–10)
76. Advanced oblique strengthening (×8–10)
71. Abdominal crunch (×6–8)
35. Upper back strengthening (×3–4)
57. Sacro-iliac joint strengthening (×4–5)
70. Straight leg sit-up (×4–5). Work slowly through full range with starting position, lying supine, hands outstretched above the head. Slowly bring the hands forwards first, then curl chin on chest and roll upwards. Finish by stretching forwards and placing the hands over the feet. Hold for 6–10 seconds, then slowly uncurl to lying position again, controlling with the abdominals all the way back down. Do *not* let the back arch.

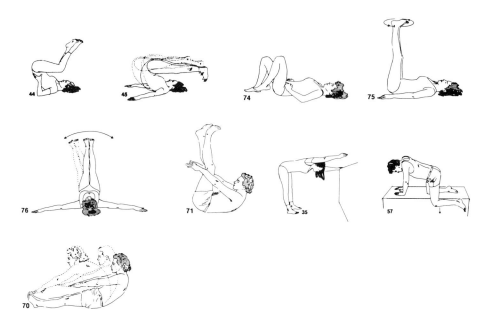

Stretches

36. Cat stretch: extension (×2–3)
37. Cat stretch: flexion (×2–3)
39. Spinal flexion/extension stretch (×2–3)
32. Latissimus dorsi/quadratus lumborum stretch (×2–3)
43. Advanced lower back stretch with hip rotation (hold for 6–10 secs, ×2–3)

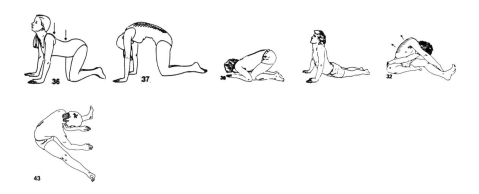

POSTURAL TYPES

The following exercise routines are designed for the five postural types which need correction: lordosis, kyphosis/lordosis, flat back, sway back and military.

When you begin your exercises it is best to practise them as often as possible — even twice daily is not excessive. However, after the first week you can reduce this amount. The minimum number of times to do the exercises is three sessions per week. Less than this and you will not see any significant changes. Ideally, it is most effective to exercise daily. The good news is that no matter what your age, you can still change your posture, though progress will be a little slower if you are over 40.

The number of times you repeat an exercise depends on how long you have neglected your body for and how keen you are to achieve results. For the strengthening exercises a basic guideline is to start off with four to five repetitions. When this becomes too easy, progress to ten. Then progress to fifteen and so on. The key to these exercises is quality and not quantity. If you cannot feel the specified area working when you are doing an exercise, review your technique — your body may be taking the easy way out and doing it incorrectly.

For the stretches, the key is to hold the stretch for about 6–10 seconds then move into the stretch a little further, repeating this two to three times. Do not bounce with your stretches. (See Chapter 2 — stretching.)

Basically, though, you are the best judge of how often you need to practise the exercises. If you do not feel or see visible improvement in your body in the short or long term, then something you are doing is wrong and you should consult a specialist.

Lordosis

73. Beginners' lower abdominals strengthening
74. Intermediate lower abdominals strengthening
68. Alternate cycling exercise
78. Adductor stretch and oblique strengthening
75. Advanced lower abdominals strengthening
63. Hip strengthening
64. Lateral rotators strengthening of the hip
37. Cat stretch: flexion
80. Adductor stretch: standing/squatting
86. Hip flexor stretch: kneeling
85. Quadriceps stretch and hip mobility: lying
38. Lower back release
48. Pelvis and lower back release

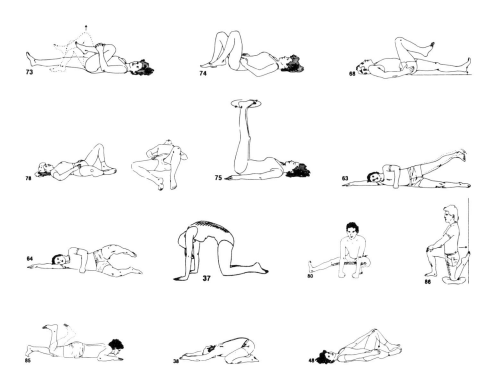

Kyphosis/lordosis

  6. Wall exercise
  1. Neck flexion
  2. Neck extension
  3. Neck rotation
  4. Neck side flexion
17. Thoracic spine and shoulder mobility exercise
18. Thoracic spine and shoulder mobility exercise with rod
19. Shoulder and scapula mobility
32. Latissimus dorsi/quadratus lumborum stretch
33. Side trunk stretch
23. Shoulder rotations: sitting
24. Shoulder rotations: lying
28. Thoracic spine and rhomboids stretch
34. Advanced thoracic spine mobility
35. Upper back strengthening
73. Beginners' lower abdominals strengthening
74. Intermediate lower abdominals strengthening
68. Alternate cycling
78. Adductor stretch and oblique strengthening
75. Advanced lower abdominals strengthening
63. Hip strengthening
64. Lateral rotators strengthening of the hip
36. Cat stretch: extension
37. Cat stretch: flexion
80. Adductor stretch: standing/squatting
84. Quadriceps stretch
38. Lower back release
48. Pelvis and lower back release

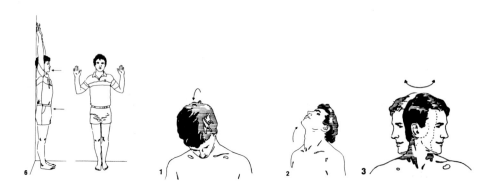

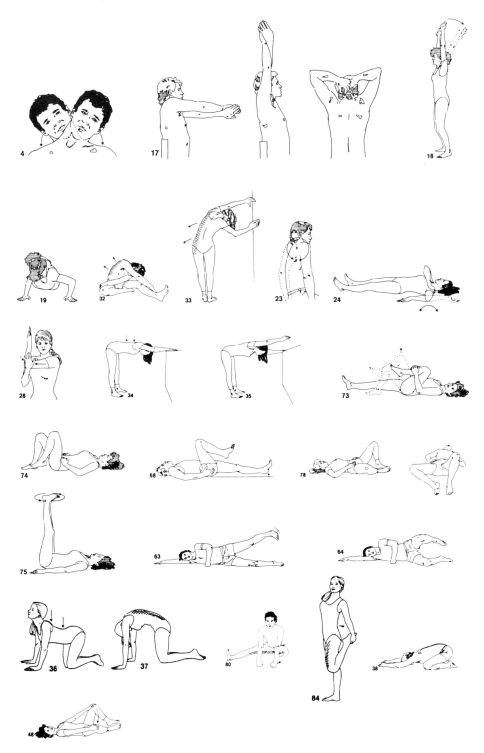

Flat back

  6. Wall exercise
  1. Neck flexion
  2. Neck extension
  3. Neck rotation
  4. Neck side flexion
 34. Advanced thoracic spine mobility
 35. Upper back strengthening
 93. Hamstring stretch: sitting
 73. Beginners' lower abdominals strengthening
 74. Intermediate lower abdominals strengthening
 78. Adductor stretch and oblique strengthening
 36. Cat stretch: extension
 37. Cat stretch: flexion
 65. Buttock strengthening
 38. Lower back release

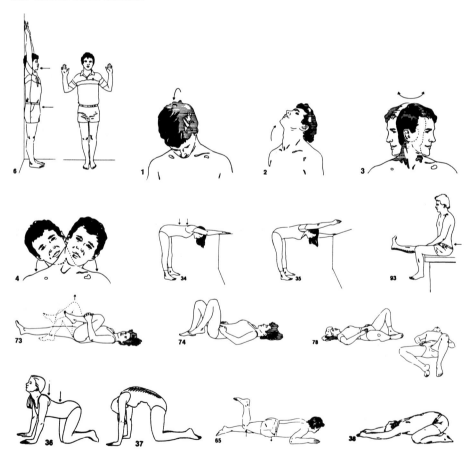

Sway back

6. Wall exercise
73. Beginners' lower abdominals strengthening
74. Intermediate lower abdominals strengthening
68. Alternate cycling
78. Adductor stretch and oblique strengthening
75. Advanced lower abdominals strengthening
76. Advanced oblique strengthening
93. Hamstring stretch: sitting
87. Hip flexor strengthening
34. Advanced thoracic spine mobility
35. Upper back strengthening
63. Hip strengthening
64. Lateral rotators strengthening of the hip
38. Lower back release

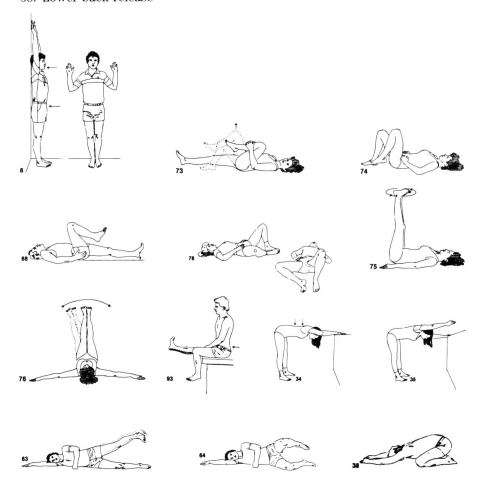

Military

6. Wall exercise
1. Neck flexion
2. Neck extension
3. Neck rotation
4. Neck side flexion
32. Latissimus dorsi/quadratus lumborum stretch
33. Side trunk stretch
35. Upper back strengthening
34. Advanced thoracic spine mobility
29. Upper back stretch
73. Beginners' lower abdominals strengthening
74. Intermediate lower abdominals strengthening
68. Alternate cycling
78. Adductor stretch and oblique strengthening
93. Hamstring stretch: sitting
44. Spinal stretch and abdominals strengthening: bent leg
45. Advanced spinal stretch and abdominals strengthening: straight leg
36. Cat stretch: extension
37. Cat stretch: flexion
19. Shoulder and scapula mobility
38. Lower back release

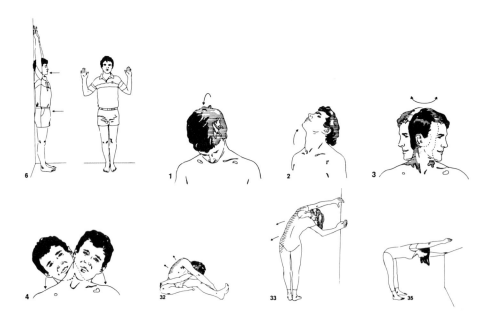

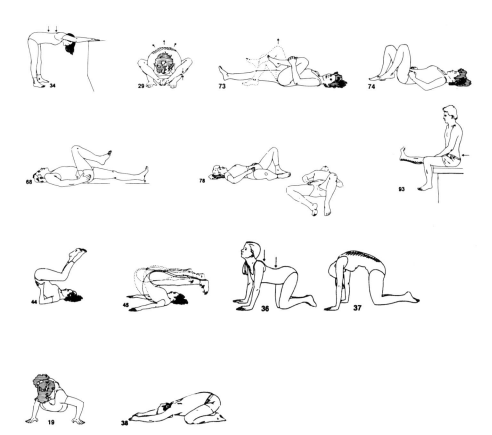

8 — EXERCISES FOR SPECIFIC SPORTS

This chapter will focus on the most commonly played sports and physical activities in our community and review special regimes for each sport, including appropriate warm-ups and cool-downs, and exercises. It must be noted that for most sports, all muscles are engaged, but each activity stresses some joints and muscles more than others. These are the areas that require additional attention.

Each diagram illustrating the sports shows the areas most vulnerable to injury. Areas of the body are numbered according to frequency of injury. For example, in football, knees are the commonest site of injury so this is marked as 1. Ankles are the next most commonly injured, so this is 2, and so on.

Pay particular attention to these areas in your stretching and warm-up as well as in your training. To gain the maximum benefit from this chapter, be sure to read the specific recommendations for your postural type, outlined in Chapter 3. If you feel you have ideal posture, then practise the exercises appropriate for your current level of fitness, in Chapter 6 — Daily routines. These exercises will ensure you retain this state of structural balance.

Not only can the exercises be performed prior to and at the end of a session of your sport, or in between sessions, but they are designed so they may be used for your daily maintenance programme. The exception to this is the section on aerobics which shows warm-up and cool-down exercises. Due to the nature of this activity, these before and after routines differ slightly.

Some of the more commonly asked questions for each sport will be addressed and answers provided. The most popular sports will be covered more comprehensively than others — aerobics, cycling, jogging, netball, walking, swimming and football — as the answers provided in these sections are relevant to all sports.

At the end of each sport a checklist will be provided. This will include the key measures you need to take to prevent injury in your sport. If the sport or activity you do is not listed here, you could devise your own checklist using the following guidelines.

SPORT CHECKLIST

Environment What is the surface or terrain like that you are exercising on? Is it easy on the body? Are you always running on uneven camber when jogging?

Equipment Have you got the most appropriate, supportive and effective equipment for your sport? (Do you have the most suitable clothing for hot weather/cold weather exercising, the correct shoes, the correct sized tennis racquet?)

The sport Have you developed the correct technique for your chosen sport? It is never too late to take lessons and get some coaching.

The individual Have you adequately warmed-up and prepared your body for the particular needs of your sport? Do you have any musculoskeletal imbalances (such as leg length difference or flat feet) that you should see a specialist about? Have you mentally prepared your mind and body for the activity you are about to undertake, particularly if you are participating in competition?

TRAINING TIPS

Not only should you take care of your muscles when you are involved in sport but you must also take care of all the skills required to be a competent player. If you have not prepared your body for the specific demands required in your sport, injury may result. Refer to Chapter 4 for general and specific training tips.

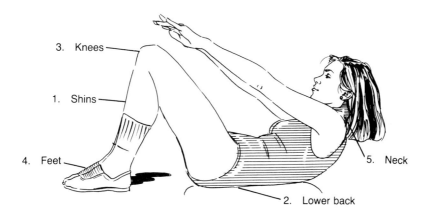

3. Knees
1. Shins
4. Feet
5. Neck
2. Lower back

AEROBICS

The past decade has seen a marked upsurge of interest in exercising to music, more commonly termed 'aerobics'. Ironically, many classes are not truly aerobic (see Chapter 2), but are anaerobic because of the high intensity level they are conducted at. Nonetheless, aerobics is an excellent means of developing all-round fitness.

The ideal fitness class is one which not only works the participants aerobically for a minimum of 25–30 minutes, but also includes stretching and strengthening of all body parts. Co-ordination and agility skills should also be included.

Aerobics can be an excellent form of exercising for all age groups provided the necessary precautions to prevent injury are taken. It is an ideal adjunct to other sports where training is often non-specific and does not concentrate on all aspects of fitness. (For instance, classes are to be highly recommended prior to football training.) The static and dynamic flexibility work, the agility and co-ordination skills, as well as the strength training incorporated in the class, far exceeds the inappropriate workouts of sit-ups and push-ups so often considered the norm preceding training in past years. The enjoyment of almost all other sports will be enhanced by the benefits gained from aerobic dance.

Common injuries

Alongside the increase in numbers in class participation, there has also been an unnecessarily high increase in injuries from aerobic dance.

Doctor James Garrick, in his report on aerobic dance in the United States, in the book *Dance Medicine*, quotes three research papers, all of which indicate the following. The commonest sites of injuries in aerobic dance listed in order of frequency of occurrence, from most common to least common are: leg/calf/achilles, knee, foot, spine, ankle, hip, other.

While the accuracy of such data is questionable, as the number of years a person had participated in classes and how many classes they were doing were omitted, the studies do support what is being seen in Australia.

The most common injuries, found clinically, are still lower limb problems (more commonly referred to as shin splints), and knee pain (usually related to the knee-cap itself). Lower back problems, clunking hips and shoulder tendonitis are the next most common complaints.

With the trend towards low-impact aerobics (minimal jumping), hopefully the incidence of high-impact (with a lot of jumping) related injuries should reduce. Nevertheless, many forms of aerobic dance still incorporate excessive jumping and high-impact work predisposing both the participant and instructor to injury.

Reasons for injury in aerobic dance

Aerobic dance currently exists in many forms. Some programmes have been heavily influenced by the instructor's jazz or ballet background. Others are more purely athletic, while some use wrist and ankle weights or rubber bands to increase the intensity of the workout. More recently, many programmes have incorporated low-impact work and high-impact jumping work is kept to a minimum.

One of the commonest reasons for injury in classes is because participants may be returning to a fitness activity after a break from exercise. They may not have the strength, flexibility or control in their bodies as they did previously, but they still try to keep up with the fitness instructor.

The key to reducing risk, if you are just commencing classes, is to choose one appropriate for your level of fitness. Most gymnasiums offer stretch and tone, or different levels of classes, to try to cater for all levels of fitness. Try to establish which class suits your current level of fitness, and build up gradually to the more advanced classes.

Many classes may still reinforce your strengths and neglect your weaknesses as everybody is put through the same regime. Be sure to assess your posture and determine what the ideal exercises are for your body type and this will help you modify those exercises which are not good for your body. (See Chapter 3.)

Commonly asked questions

Are instructors' injuries the same as participants'?

The site of injury is usually the same for both groups (the lower limb, the back and the hips). What differs is usually in the number of classes instructors need to take each week. Also, when they do get an injury, because classes are often their sole source of income, they are rarely able to rest to let it heal.

Overuse injuries, particularly shin pain, and often stress fractures, are not un-common amongst instructors. How many classes an instructor takes each week is purely individual, but not more than seven to nine advanced classes per week is advisable.

Another factor influencing instructors' injuries is their background. If this has been one of dance or gymnastics they will tend to be very flexible in all their joints. If this is not balanced out by appropriate strengthening and proprioceptive (balance) work, instability around joints is likely to occur, leading to overuse problems in the long term.

Is there an ideal aerobic shoe?

The answer to date is, no. However, many shoes are adequate. One of the prob-lems is to design a shoe that can withstand full body weight and shock both on the forefoot, and on both the medial and the lateral aspect of the foot. That is, multi-directional support is required.

Jogging is a predominantly unidirectional activity, so sometimes jogging shoes can be risky, with all the change of direction activity required in the class, because of their broad base (see Jogging). Tennis or squash shoes, designed for agility, often lack forefoot stability and back foot support.

Therefore, it is a matter of finding a shoe that meets your requirements. Most shoes given the label 'aerobic', attempt to cater for the complex needs required in aerobic dance. The key factors to look for are: adequate heel support and arch support, forefoot support for lateral stability, flexibility in the forefoot — does it come in the right place for your foot — and so on.

Some of the most recently produced shoes cater for the above. If you are an instructor be sure to review, and maybe replace, your shoes every three to four months.

Checklist

Make sure the fitness instructor has taken some form of accredited instructor training.

Make sure the class is suitable to your level of fitness.

The structure of the class should include warm-up, strengthening for all major muscle groups, an aerobic component and a cool-down.

Check the floor surface is not too jarring for your body. Concrete floors covered with carpet are particularly stressful for the lower limb.

Ensure you have adequately supportive aerobic shoes.

You should not be doing too much running or jumping in the one direction — particularly if you are currently overweight. If your shins are sore, then maybe you are doing too much jumping.

If you come from a dancing background, try to incorporate at least one dance class a week to regain your balance, appropriate for your degree of flexibility.

Look at yourself when working out at the gym, in mirrors provided, to see if you need to improve your form and technique when doing each exercise.

Be careful not to attend, or take, too many classes. Overuse injuries are a sure sign you are doing too many classes for your body.

Watch your technique and form when exercising. High-speed, out of control movements, can result in injury.

Practise balance and control work so that excessive movements around your joints do not occur when you are landing after a jump.

Establish which exercises are beneficial for your body and those which are unsuitable. Modify these in your class.

You may need a postural assessment by a sports specialist to screen for leg length differences, bowed legs, flat feet etc.

Warm-up and cool-down: Make sure you slowly increase the pace at which you workout in a class and slowly cool-down and stretch at the completion of the class. A minimum of 8–10 minutes should be spent in both warm-up and cool-down. If you are late for a class, do your own warm-up and stretch, rather than starting straight into a high-impact workout.

Aerobics exercise routine

Warm-up

1. Neck flexion
2. Neck extension
3. Neck rotation

4. Neck side flexion
5. Neck stretch
17. Thoracic spine and shoulder mobility exercise
18. Thoracic spine and shoulder mobility exercise using a rod
23. Shoulder rotations: sitting
24. Shoulder rotations: lying
21. Tricep stretch
22. Latissimus dorsi stretch
97. Combined hamstring and adductor stretch
84. Quadriceps stretch
103. Calf stretch
104. Step stretch
106. Achilles and soleus stretch
111. Shin strengthening

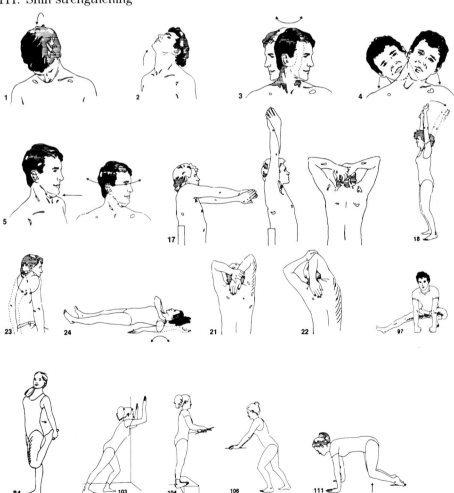

Cool-down

1. Neck flexion
2. Neck extension
3. Neck rotation
4. Neck side flexion
25. Shoulder shrugs
36. Cat stretch: extension
37. Cat stretch: flexion
59. Hip stretch for piriformis and sciatica
60. Advanced hip stretch
38. Lower back release
40. Passive back extension stretch
29. Upper back stretch
32. Latissimus dorsi/quadratus lumborum stretch
33. Side trunk stretch
41. Lower back stretch
42. Advanced lower back stretch
43. Advanced lower back stretch with hip rotation
49. Knee hug stretch
99. Upper hamstring stretch: lying
50. Spinal rotation stretch: lying
51. Double leg spinal rotation
52. Spinal rotation stretch: sitting
48. Pelvis and lower back release

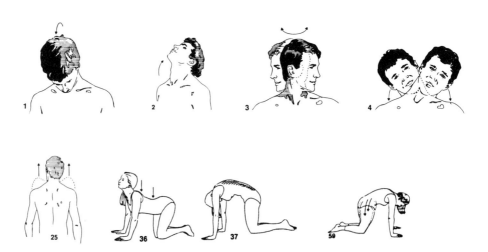

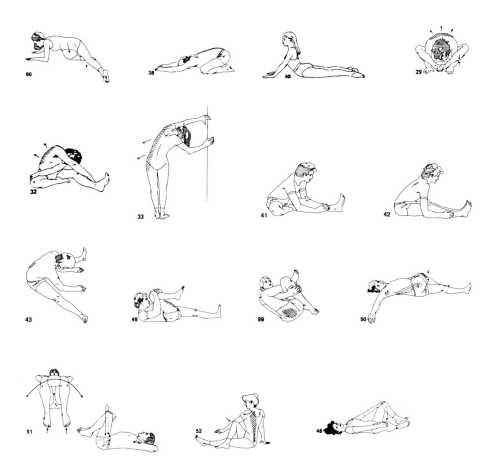

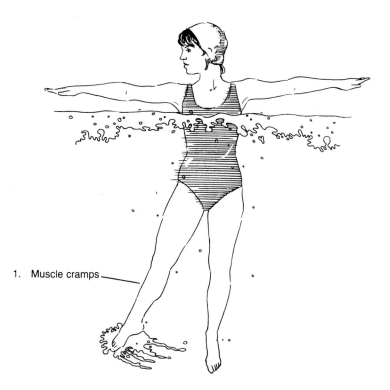

1. Muscle cramps

AQUAROBICS

Exercising to music in the water is a fun activity and is suitable for all age groups. Because of the decreased load on weight-bearing joints, injuries should be minimal. The only regular complaint is that of calf cramps. Adequate stretching, prior to working in the water, can minimise this. Also, try not to land on the toes but 'through the foot' in the water. Trauma, due to slipping beside the pool, sometimes occurs. This can be avoided if adequate precautions are taken.

Advantages of aquarobics

- It is suitable for all ages, and in particular, is ideal for the elderly.
- For the overweight, it provides minimal stress on weight-bearing joints and less self-consciousness while they workout.
- One can work all joints throughout their full range with resistance (of the water).
- It is suitable for those with chronic back complaints, arthritis and other similar musculoskeletal disorders.
- Being able to swim is not an essential prerequisite to enjoy aquarobics safely.
- It is suitable for athletes when they have injuries aggravated by weight-bearing activities (such as sprinters or marathon runners).
- It is suitable during pregnancy.

The disadvantage of aquarobics

- One can cheat in the water because it is difficult for the instructor to supervise underwater movements accurately, and full range of movement may not be performed. Therefore, the workout intensity level may be too low to be truly aerobic.

Checklist

- Pool temperature should be 25–28 degrees. For pre-natal it should definitely not be greater than 30 degrees. The ideal is 28 degrees.
- If instructing, ensure you have suitable footwear that does not permit slipping on the edge of the pool.
- Aquarobics is suitable for all ages. However, check with your doctor if you have a medical condition, particularly if you have high blood pressure and are unsure if aquarobics is suitable for you.
- Be careful not to jump on your toes in the pool. Land through the whole foot to avoid leg cramps.
- Be sure to work all muscles through their full range.
- If feeling faint at any time let the instructor know immediately.
- Try not to compromise movements and work the body through its full range.

Warm-up and cool-down: A minimum of 8–10 minutes should be allocated for each. Warm-up and stretches can be done either in or out of the pool. Partner stretches are ideal for cool-down. Using the walls at the edge of the pool can also make stretching more effective.

Aquarobics exercise routine

1. Neck flexion
2. Neck extension
3. Neck rotation
4. Neck side flexion
5. Neck stretch to correct a lordotic cervical spine
17. Thoracic spine and shoulder mobility exercise
21. Tricep stretch
22. Latissimus dorsi stretch
33. Side trunk stretch
97. Combined hamstring and adductor stretch
18. Thoracic spine and shoulder mobility exercise using a rod
84. Quadriceps stretch
103. Calf stretch
105. Combined gastrocnemius/peroneal stretch
106. Achilles and soleus stretch
117. Ankle mobility

Some of these stretches may be performed while in the pool, using the edge of the pool to assist with the stretches.

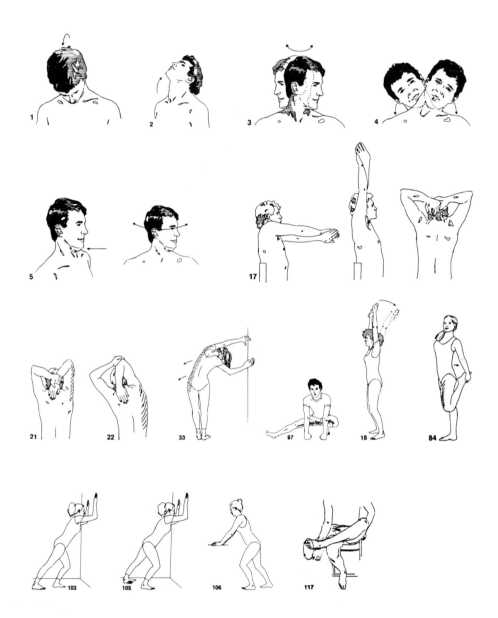

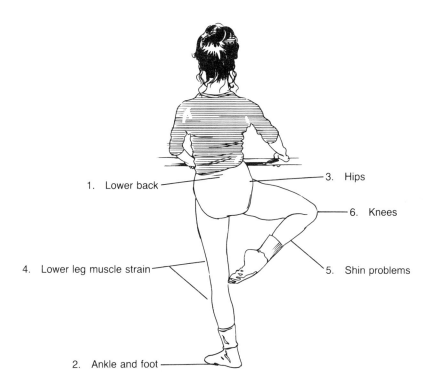

1. Lower back

3. Hips

6. Knees

4. Lower leg muscle strain

5. Shin problems

2. Ankle and foot

BALLET AND GYMNASTICS

While many take up ballet in their younger years, only a select few continue to dance recreationally in later years, and even fewer dance professionally.

Many dancers participate in other forms of dance besides classical ballet, such as jazz and modern dance. Traditionally though, a child is introduced to classical ballet when she or he first starts to dance.

On a professional level we tend to think of dancers as artists. Yet the degree of athletic competence required by dancers readily equals that of any sport. A typical work schedule during a season for a professional ballet dancer often includes 9 hours in class, 26 hours in rehearsal and 8–12 hours in performance, for a total of 43–48 hours during a 6 day period. (Ryan and Stephens, *Dance Medicine*, page 7.) Dance students, while in training, often practise up to 8 hours per day. Fortunately, the medical and paramedical fraternity are starting to recognise the demands placed on the dancer's body and to meet the needs accordingly. Rest is usually not the appropriate solution to treating a dancer's injury. (However, it is not the intent of this book to discuss the élite athlete as this is another topic.)

On a recreational level, dance injuries are usually few in number, probably because those participating in dance classes only participate in three to four classes per week and they do not use this as their sole form of fitness but balance this activity with other sports.

Dance classes are an excellent means of maintaining suppleness, increasing strength and even improving posture because of the control and poise encouraged when each movement is executed.

Most of the key factors concerning gymnastics are similar to those of dance. On a professional level the demands on the body are great. Regular massage and always stretching and strengthening the body through full range is to be highly recommended.

On a recreational level the concern focuses around children as only a select few continue with gymnastics beyond their 20s and, if they do so, should be working closely with a coach.

For children excessive jumping and lower back hyperextension should not be forced or performed in high repetition in the years of 5–11. As the ligaments start to mature beyond this age, and muscle strength starts to develop, attention to control and balance around joints is imperative. If possible, children, no matter what age, should combine gymnastics with other forms of sport. When children are going through a growth spurt, training should be eased back a little. Two to three times per week is sufficient training for a child to perform gymnastics on a recreational basis.

The main injuries from gymnastics relate to the development of an excessive lumbar lordosis. Unfortunately, this is a necessary part of many of the techniques performed. Maintaining strength in the lower abdominals (particularly external oblique) can reduce the risk of excessive strain of the lower back.

Commonly asked questions

Is there an ideal age for children to commence ballet or to start pointe work?

There is no harm in a child starting ballet as young as 5 years old. However, it is imperative that both teacher and parent do not push the child in the early years. As a rule, males tend to take up dance when slightly older compared with females, probably more because of social expectations than anything else. It also seems the female child is usually the one with demands placed on her beyond her years.

Before the age of 10 emphasis should be on the development of proper execution of techniques and minimal emphasis on forcing stretches (particularly turnout). A child's ligaments are immature at this age and can easily be overstretched. Emphasis on working to end of range and development of balance, control and strength throughout range should be the focus of dance classes for the child.

Dance teachers must be aware of the anatomic, technical and long term detrimental implications of forcing a child on pointe too early. Dr Ryan in his book *Dance Medicine*, states, 'pointe work should not be permitted before the age of 10 years, and should be strictly limited to a series of gradually progressive exercises between the ages of 10 and 12'.

Because the bones are growing, there are still growth plates in each bone. These are called the epiphyseal plates. This region of the bone is soft and easily damaged particularly at the base of the first or second toes. Therefore, it is critical that a child does not go up on pointe till adequate strength and control in lower limb and foot musculature is developed. For most children this may be 12–13 years old. A 1 or 2 year delay in starting full-time pointe work, providing the child is learning and practising good ballet technique, can prevent many foot problems occurring later in life.

Another point is that sometimes the parent and teacher have to acknowledge and let the child know that he or she is simply not suited to dance.

Key anatomical factors that predispose a dancer of any age to problems are:

1. Somatotype (body type and shape — see Chapter 2). Ectomorphs and mesomorph tendencies are far more suited to dance than individuals who are shorter and plumper (endomorphs).
2. Femoral angle (the angle of the femur in relation to the hip). Females with very broad hips tend to have a severe femoral angle predisposing them to injury.
3. Femoral torsion (the rotation of the femur). Because of the demand for extreme external rotation (turn-out) femoral anteversion, that is, internally rotated femurs, are not ideal for dancing.
4. Genu recurvatum (the curve of the knees from the side). This refers to hyperextension of the knees and usually leads to the dancer standing with a hyperlordosed back. A child may grow out of this skeletal type but while it is severe, the child should refrain from regular dance.
5. Tibial torsion (rotation of the tibia). Normally the tibia is externally twisted about 12 degrees along its length. Excessive external tibial torsion (greater than 20 degrees) may result in knee disorders (usually patellofemoral) because the dancer cannot align the knees over the toes during plié (when the feet and hips are turned out and the knees are flexed).
6. Foot-type. Either flat feet, a very rigid supinated foot, or bilateral bunion deformities create problems for the child dancer.

Withstanding all the above, it must be added that while anatomical factors may limit the amount and calibre of participation for the child, they should not hamper the individual's desire to dance within the limits of one's own abilities, discipline and talent, thereby providing pain-free enjoyment.

Checklist

- Floor surfaces should not be too hard. Sprung board is ideal.
- Apart from the actual gym equipment, requirements are minimal though taping to the foot directly to support minor foot disorders may be needed by some.

- Be sure the demands of training by the teacher are not too great for you as an individual.
- Try to balance dance classes with other forms of aerobic activity.
- Are you suited to ballet or gymnastics? Be realistic in your goals.
- Children should not be pushed by parent or teacher to progress beyond their skeletal age. Going up on pointe before 11 to 12 years and forcing turn-out is not recommended.
- Males interested in dance prior to their teens should be encouraged. This will prevent excessive work having to be done in later teen years.

Ballet/gymnastics exercise routine

1. Neck flexion
2. Neck extension
3. Neck rotation
4. Neck side flexion
19. Shoulder and scapula mobility
21. Tricep stretch
22. Latissimus dorsi stretch
32. Latissimus dorsi/quadratus lumborum stretch
33. Side trunk stretch
29. Upper back stretch
34. Advanced thoracic spine mobility
39. Spinal flexion/extension
41. Lower back stretch
42. Advanced lower back stretch
43. Advanced lower back stretch with hip rotation
50. Spinal rotation stretch
60. Advanced hip stretch
78. Adductor stretch and oblique strengthening
86. Hip flexor stretch
103. Calf stretch
106. Achilles and soleus stretch
107. Deep toe flexor stretch
117. Ankle mobility
116. Intrinsic foot strengthening

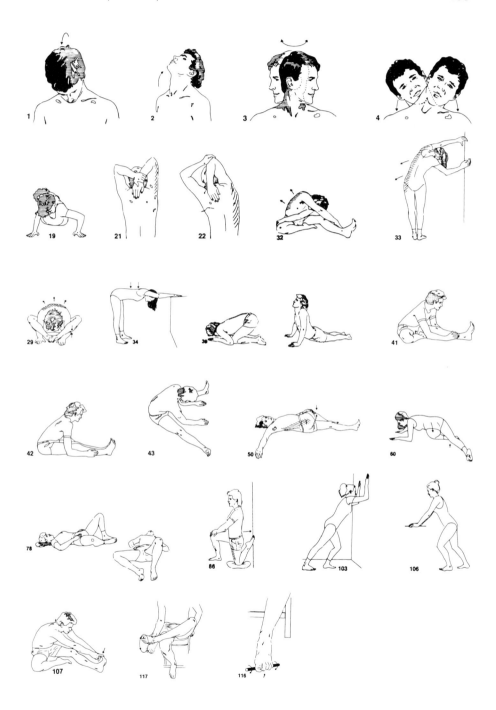

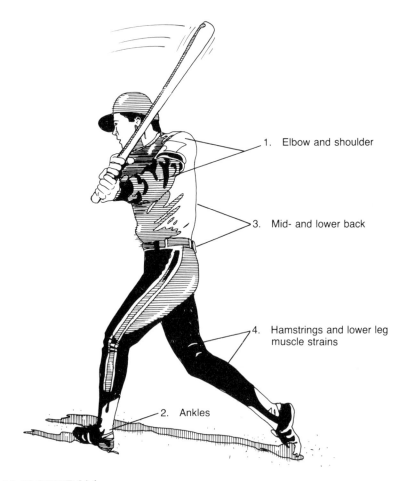

1. Elbow and shoulder

3. Mid- and lower back

4. Hamstrings and lower leg muscle strains

2. Ankles

BASEBALL/SOFTBALL

While softball has been played for many years in Australia, baseball has only become more popular in recent years. Both are predominantly anaerobic activities because of their stop/start nature. But if combined with a regular fitness programme, the enjoyment of your game will be significantly enhanced.

For both sports, injuries are usually to the elbow, shoulder, fingers, wrist and hand, to the lower back and minor traumas to the lower limb musculature, in order of frequency of occurrence.

Elbow injuries in these two sports are often termed 'pitcher's elbow'. The problem may occur on either the medial or lateral aspect of the elbow. Usually the problem starts as tendonitis (inflammation of the tendon) or bursitis (inflammation of the bursa, which is the sac that permits free riding of a tendon over a bone). If the player continues to pitch, the problem can be easily aggravated and a chronic problem may develop. Sometimes surgery is required in the more severe cases, where excess bone or calcium has been deposited, by the body, around the elbow, to protect it against the continual overload of the tendons and muscles in this area.

The most common reasons for both elbow and shoulder injuries (such as tendonitis) occurring, is usually poor technique, muscle imbalance or inflexibility around the elbow or shoulder, attempting to provide excessive spin to the ball while pitching or throwing, or simply overtraining.

A coach can assist with technique, while stretching will balance flexibility around the shoulder girdle.

Checklist

- Be sure the bat size is suited to your grip.
- Review your technique of throwing and pitching if you are getting elbow or shoulder problems.
- Warm-up well including stretching prior to practice and match play.
- Try to do some form of aerobic exercise to improve your general level of fitness.
- Warm-up slowly and do not practise throwing skills and pitching skills for extended periods of time with no break.

Warm-up: All major muscle groups need loosening prior to practice or match play. Large circular swinging movements (both forwards and backwards) of the shoulders, and a light jog around the oval should precede the following stretches. Skills such as throwing and pitching should be practised slowly at first before attempting to perform at match-play speed. Agility skills such as stop/start runs between the bases to specifically prepare the lower limb for this type of demand during match play, should also be practised.

Baseball/softball exercise routine

  17. Thoracic spine and shoulder mobility exercise
  19. Shoulder and scapula mobility
  21. Tricep stretch
  22. Latissimus dorsi stretch
  26. Wrist, shoulder and neck stretch
  30. Posterior shoulder and thoracic spine stretch
  32. Latissimus dorsi/quadratus lumborum stretch
  33. Side trunk stretch
  52. Spinal rotation stretch: sitting
  80. Adductor stretch: standing/squatting
  84. Quadriceps stretch
 103. Calf stretch
 105. Combined gastrocnemius/peroneal stretch
 106. Achilles and soleus stretch

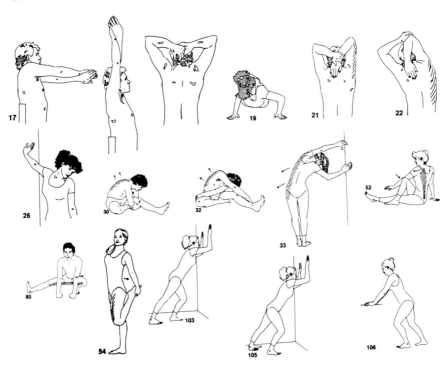

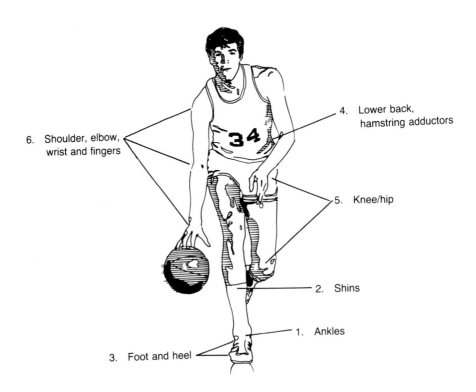

BASKETBALL

The speed at which this game is played means injury is usually due to high-impact collisions either with the hard ground or with another player. Major trauma can occur in basketball, particularly to the knees, ankles, fingers and hands, so adequate warm-up of all major muscle groups is essential. In addition, one should practise specific agility and ball and reflex skills prior to a game. Shin soreness, back and shoulder complaints are usually more related to over-training than direct trauma.

Basketball shoes

While the higher ankle shoe used in basketball definitely provides some support and stability to the ankle, a sprained ankle within the boot is still vulnerable. Therefore taping is a must to provide additional support. Balance and strengthening exercises should also be performed, using resisted exercise machines if possible. An inner tube of a bicycle or a 50–75 centimetre (20–30 inch) strip of strong elastic or rubber band is also ideal for strengthening. (See exercises 113 and 115.)

If frequency of ankle sprains continues even though exercises have been performed regularly, a strong supportive guard with velcro straps (not elastic) may be required.

The diagram below shows taping of an ankle for an inversion, that is, an inwardly turned, sprain.

Use sports tape, 4–5 centimetres (½–2 inches) width.

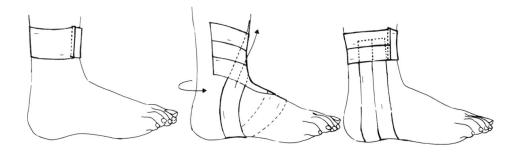

8.1   Ankle taping

Ankle taping

Step 1: Anchor straps: Place one strap at a slight angle round the circumference of the calf, just below where it joins the achilles tendon. Have the tape at the back of the leg, lower than the front. Slightly overlap the tape at the front.

Step 2 (stirrups): Place two strips of tape, starting from the inside border of the anchor strap under the foot and up onto the outside of the leg, back onto the anchor strap.

Step 3: Now place the tape on the inside of the leg and pull up and out. (See Figure 8.1.) Pull the foot into eversion and keep the ankle at right angles. Finish this tape across the front of the ankle. Use three strips of tape here — each overlapping slightly.

Step 4: Finish off the taping by putting strips around the ankle to secure the tape. Leave a slight gap where the tape meets in case of swelling.

Checklist

- Try to train on a variety of surfaces if possible.
- Be sure to wear appropriate and supportive footwear. Wear basketball boots if possible. Wear ankle or finger taping (see Netball) or a guard if carrying an injury, or for prevention purposes, post-injury.
- The skills required for this sport include a basic level of aerobic and anaerobic fitness as well as balance, co-ordination and agility. Ball skills, and good jumping technique are also required.
- Practise the skills for your specific position of play. Ensure you have practised shooting goals both close to and at wider range. If you are getting symptoms such as shin splints, reassess your training programme (you may be over-training). Also review your feet for faulty mechanics. Adequate warm-up, stretching and practice of ball skills prior to a match are critical. Jumping practice for basketball is essential. Plyometrics can assist this. This refers to using a muscle eccentrically, then performing a concentric contraction as soon as possible after the first contraction. An example would be jumping off a box onto the ground then jumping straight up onto another box. This would be plyometric training for the quadriceps. The aim of plyometrics is to improve one's jumping skills, and is recommended for all sports where jumping is required.

Warm-up: A light jog around the basketball court followed by specific stretching with focus on the ankles, calves, hamstrings, lower back and shoulder and torso musculature is essential. Practising specific ball catching while moving, agility skills (side-stepping, shuttle sprints slowly increasing the pace) and goal-shooting by all players, after stretching, must be incorporated in the warm-up.

Basketball exercise routine

17. Thoracic spine and shoulder mobility exercise
32. Latissimus dorsi/quadratus lumborum stretch
33. Side trunk stretch
21. Tricep stretch
22. Latissimus dorsi stretch
34. Advanced thoracic spine mobility
30. Posterior shoulder and thoracic spine stretch
97. Combined hamstring and adductor stretch
44. Spinal stretch and abdominals strengthening
103. Calf stretch
105. Combined gastrocnemius/peroneal stretch
106. Achilles and soleus stretch
84. Quadriceps stretch
111. Shin strengthening
19. Shoulder and scapula mobility

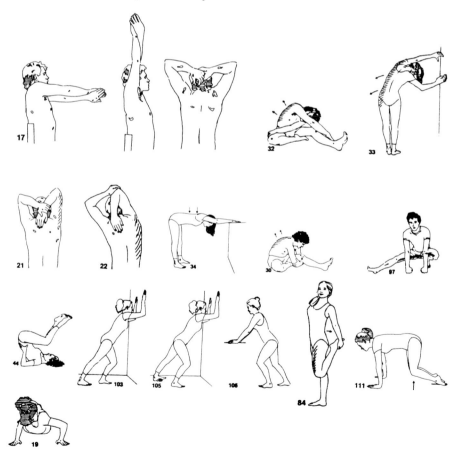

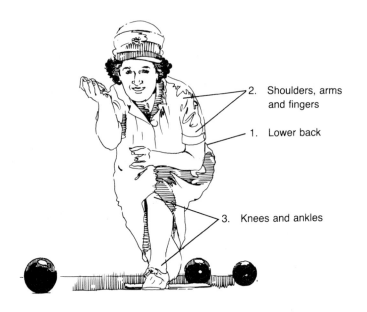

2. Shoulders, arms and fingers

1. Lower back

3. Knees and ankles

BOWLING

Lawn bowls would appear at first glance to be a relatively injury free activity, because of the age group who adopt this activity. However, as we become older, precautionary measures are a must.

Lawn bowls is not only an excellent social outing for those who participate regularly, but is also an excellent means of keeping the body supple and co-ordinated — particularly in the later years. Even if no previous regular exercise has been undertaken, providing a few basic precautions are observed, bowls should be a safe form of physical activity for anyone.

One of the potential problem areas in bowls can be the lower back. The most stressful position for the discs, ligaments and muscles of the lower back is in flexion (bending forward) and rotation. Good technique by bending directly over the bent knee keeping the spine quite straight, trying not to bend forward from just the neck, shoulders and upper back, should prevent this potentially stressful position. Nonetheless, if you play bowls regularly, or even if you do so infrequently, the following stretches and tips will reduce your chance of aches or pains at the end of a day of bowls or the next day. It must be remembered though that bowls is not an effective form of aerobic exercise. It should be combined with other weekly activities such as swimming or brisk walking.

Ten pin bowls is predominantly a fun activity. It requires minimal warm-up, but a few stretches prior to playing can reduce the risk of overstraining a muscle.

Checklist

- Always include a warm-up prior to a game, and review your technique regularly.
- Try to walk to the bowling green to loosen up joints and muscles prior to a game.

Warm-up: Take deep breaths in while loosening up the shoulders and arms with slow circular movements. Give special attention to the calves, quadriceps, hamstrings, lower back, shoulders, forearms and fingers in your stretches.

- Do not wait to be stiff in your joints and muscles after bowling.
- Do stretches nightly for 8–10 minutes (minimum) in between games as well as prior to your sport. Your extra suppleness will enhance the enjoyment of your game.
- Loosen the fingers and wrist prior to commencing play.

Bowling exercise routine

1. Neck flexion
2. Neck extension
3. Neck rotation
4. Neck side flexion
17. Thoracic spine and shoulder mobility exercise
25. Shoulder shrugs
26. Wrist, shoulder and neck stretch
27. Wrist and finger stretch
28. Thoracic spine and rhomboids stretch
21. Tricep stretch
22. Latissimus dorsi stretch
33. Side trunk stretch
36. Cat stretch: extension
37. Cat stretch: flexion
38. Lower back release
41. Lower back stretch
80. Adductor stretch: standing/squatting (do not do full squat position)
78. Adductor stretch and oblique strengthening
84. Quadriceps stretch
85. Quadriceps stretch and hip mobility: lying
98. Upper hamstring stretch
103. Calf stretch
105. Combined gastrocnemius/peroneal stretch
106. Achilles and soleus stretch
117. Ankle mobility

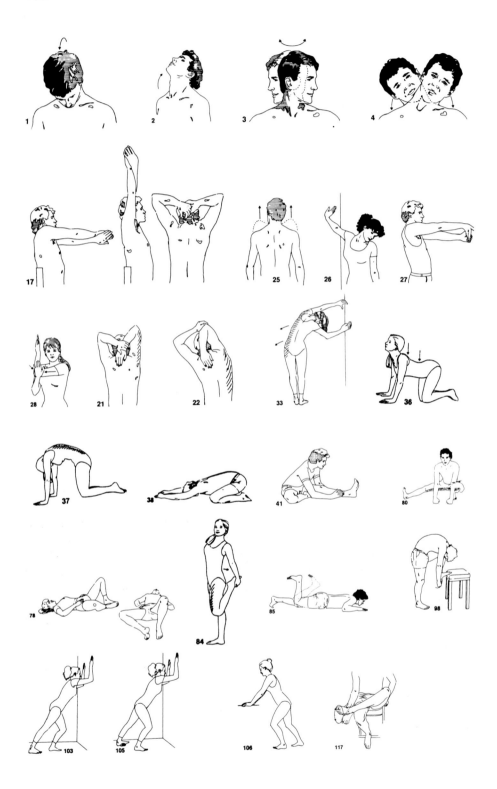

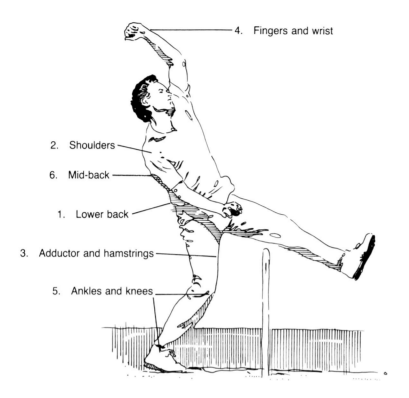

4. Fingers and wrist

2. Shoulders

6. Mid-back

1. Lower back

3. Adductor and hamstrings

5. Ankles and knees

CRICKET

The skills required for a game of cricket are varied. On a social level injury is usually due to inadequate or inappropriate skill training, while at grade, advanced or first-grade level, injury is usually due to overtraining. On both levels, however, the time spent either waiting in outer field or waiting to bat poses the biggest problem. When the body does have to move to field a ball or to go out and bat, the intensity and level of activity required is usually high-speed and sudden, on a body that has been inactive for some time. This can cause problems.

Because of the intermittent nature of the game for some players and the infrequency of their training or playing cricket, muscle strains of the shoulder, back or forearm occur too often, even during social games. At other levels, shoulder tendonitis and back problems due to overtraining or poor throwing or bowling technique are the most frequently occurring injuries. Foot, hip and knee problems may occur for these same reasons.

A good preventative measure is to keep moving if you are fielding in the outer boundaries. Doing leg stretches and keeping the arms loose and stretched should be possible without distracting the batter!

Other measures include reviewing your bowling and throwing technique, by getting a coach to look at your style and form. Social cricketers often do not train between weekly matches or worse still go down to the cricket nets once per week to do an hour or more of just practice bowling — no warm-up, no stretch! No matter what level you play, it is advisable not to spend more than half an hour at any one time practising just bowling without a break. Include some stretching during your break periods.

Breaks from repetitively practising skills are even more important for the élite player, as many more hours are usually spent in overall training. Because of this, individual body mechanics, flexibility and strength, in addition to bowling or throwing technique, are even more important.

Commonly asked questions

Why do so many fast bowlers get back pain?

There is a direct relationship between the particular technique used for bowling and the incidence of lower back pain. Bowlers who land with the foot they plant with, in too much of an internally rotated position, create additional stress through their knees, hips and backs. The extended and rotated position the back is in when the foot is planted causes excessive overstressing of all spinal structures. A foot rotated too far internally means the spine must extend and rotate even further to achieve follow-through and to provide speed and power in the throw. The ideal position is to have the planted foot such that the outside (lateral) border of the foot is directly adjacent and parallel to the crease. This reduces the stress on the lower back.

Are the stresses in indoor cricket similar to outdoor?

Indoor cricket is quite different to outdoor. The pace is faster, agility skills are more essential because of the confined space it is played in, and injuries are often of a more traumatic nature. Impact injuries with either other players or the ground are not uncommon. Aside from this, the rules for the eight players and preventative measures, including review of technique, adequate training and warm-up and specific skills practised prior to play are still essential. Time to cool-down and tighten up in the muscles while playing is certainly not a factor contributing to injury in indoor cricket.

Checklist

- Always wear supportive shoes.
- Do you get back, shoulder pain after playing? Review your bowling or throwing technique if you do.
- Are you doing practice sessions between matches? Do you warm-up slowly

prior to a match or training? Take rest breaks when practising bowling, a minimum of one every half hour, and include some stretching in the breaks.

Warm-up: The ultimate will be when we see our top grade players going for a jog round the oval prior to a match! Occasionally it is seen in top level cricket, but certainly not enough. Ideally, before a match, all players should warm-up all major muscle groups, particularly the shoulders, back, adductors (groin muscles), and hamstrings should be adequately stretched. While fielding in outer field try to keep moving and if getting ready to bat go through the following stretches again. Before fielding be sure to practise throwing and do some bowling, slowly building up your pace.

Cricket exercise routine

17. Thoracic spine and shoulder mobility exercise
26. Wrist, shoulder and neck stretch
27. Wrist and finger stretch
21. Tricep stretch
22. Latissimus dorsi stretch
11. Pectoral stretch
31. Posterior shoulder and upper back stretch
33. Side trunk stretch
41. Lower back stretch
32. Latissimus dorsi/quadratus lumborum stretch
80. Adductor stretch: standing/squatting
81. Adductor stretch: sitting
49. Knee hug stretch
84. Quadriceps stretch
61. Hip abductor stretch *OR*
62. Advanced hip abductor stretch
103. Calf stretch
105. Combined gastrocnemius/peroneal stretch
106. Achilles and soleus stretch
52. Spinal rotation stretch: sitting

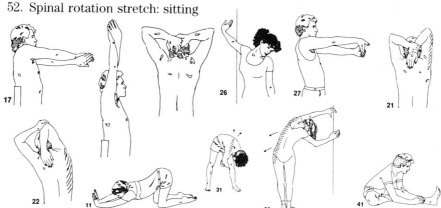

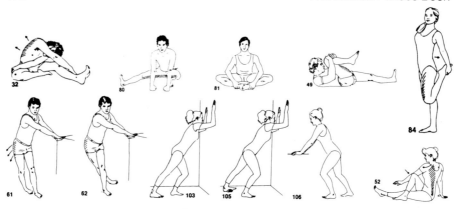

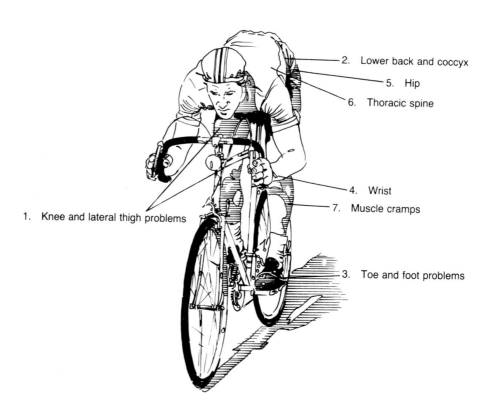

2. Lower back and coccyx

5. Hip

6. Thoracic spine

4. Wrist

7. Muscle cramps

1. Knee and lateral thigh problems

3. Toe and foot problems

CYCLING

Whether you cycle as your sole form of fitness or as part of your weekly fitness programme, cycling is only partially weight-bearing, so its stress on the body should be minimal.

Injuries in cycling usually affect the knees, back, wrist, forearms or neck. Cramps in the calves or thighs are also common. Trying to vary your position while you are actually cycling, such as arching the back in, then out again, or stretching the hands, can reduce the stiffness that can set in on a long ride.

The most important consideration in cycling is to choose a bike suited to your individual needs. Ideally have your bike custom made if you can. The following are the basic recommendations for choosing a bicycle.

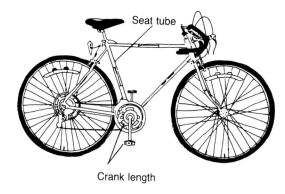

8.2   Bicycle

The bike

There are eight key factors to consider when choosing and setting up your bike. These are:

1. *Frame size.* Choosing a bike appropriate for your height and size is essential to minimise injury risk. Correct frame size is determined by the length of the seat tube (see Figure 8.2). This measurement is equal to the inside leg length, minus twice the crank length.
2. *Saddle height.* Seated on the bicycle with heels on pedals (wearing cycling shoes if you use these in training), the legs should be bent slightly at the bottom of the arc when pedalling backwards, without causing the pelvis to move.
3. *Seat angle.* This should be level with the top bar of the frame, or the nose can be slightly tilted up.
4. *Handlebar position.* The body should lean forward so that the eye level is over the middle of the front wheel. The mountain bike, which has seen an increase in popularity in recent years, permits the body to be more upright. This places less load on the back, because its handlebars are in a more upright position.
5. *Head stem length.* While the top bar length is usually custom made for each size bike, the head stem length can be altered. Elbows should be slightly bent and comfortable, not outstretched, if this readjustment is made.
6. *Cleats.* These should be positioned on the mid-line at the base of the first to fifth metatarsals, right in the centre, that is, so that the ball of the foot is over the pedal axle.
7. *Toe straps and toe clips.* These improve the efficiency of your cycling by permitting work to be done as the leg moves up as well as when it pushes down.

8. *Gear ratios.* If you work in a gear that provides too much resistance unnecessarily to your legs, you will fatigue easily and be prone to injury. The ideal is to pedal at a rate of approximately 80–100 revolutions per minute. This is the most efficient rate on any terrain which provides least resistance on the body. Therefore, when you change gears, you should still be pedalling around this rate. If you are unfit, the rate is 70–100 revolutions per minute. For the fitter it is 80–100. This can be easily calculated while riding by counting revolutions over 15 seconds and multiplying by four. Learning to use your gears correctly can also make riding more enjoyable and efficient.

Stationary bicycles

In some ways stationary bicycles can be much more effective than road bikes because it is safe within the confines of their space to increase their pace as much as you need to work aerobically. Be sure to monitor your pulse rate if you are using the bike as your means of aerobically keeping fit and try to maintain the cycling for 20–30 minutes. To prevent muscle stiffness stretch before and after your workout.

The main drawbacks of the stationary bikes is their short term interest by the owner. If one could afford both types of bikes, this would be ideal. Then with inclement weather the stationary bike can be used and on other days one can still cycle outside.

Checklist

- As you cycle get a friend to watch you from behind and see if your foot or knee turns inward as you cycle. You may need orthotics in your shoes or have a muscle imbalance around your hip if you have too much rotation in your leg movement. Consult a sports specialist to correct this.
- When going up a hill, lean forward if you need to rise off the seat. This will give you greater power.
- Learn to use your gears correctly to reduce the stress on your legs and to have a more efficient ride.
- It is very easy to gain minimal aerobic fitness from cycling, so if it is your sole form of fitness be sure to push yourself to increase your heart rate appropriately. If you live in the city you may need to allocate days where you try to get to a park where you can safely increase your pace.
- Try to introduce hills in your cycle to increase the aerobic effectiveness of your workout.
- Review the guidelines listed to be sure your bike is suited to your specific needs.
- Adjust the seat, the handlebars, the cleats and the pressure in your tyres to suit the roads you are cycling on.
- If cycling is your sole form of fitness be sure you are working at an effective aerobic intensity for your age.

- Cycling is ideal to balance with walking, swimming or jogging. If your back aches after you cycle, check your handlebars are not too low, or too far forward. For touring, and outback exploring, consider investing in a mountain bike.
- Do you stand with knock-knees or do you have excessively flat feet? Consult a sports specialist or podiatrist if you do, particularly if you are getting any pain in the lower limbs when you cycle, as this may be your predisposition.

Cycling exercise routine

17. Thoracic spine and shoulder mobility exercise
21. Tricep stretch
22. Latissimus dorsi stretch
26. Wrist, shoulder and neck stretch
27. Wrist and finger stretch
34. Advanced thoracic spine mobility
33. Side trunk stretch
32. Latissimus dorsi/quadratus lumborum stretch
36. Cat stretch: extension
37. Cat stretch: flexion
38. Lower back release
49. Knee hug stretch
61. Hip abductor stretch *OR*
62. Advanced hip abductor stretch
80. Adductor stretch: standing/squatting
78. Adductor stretch and oblique strengthening
84. Quadriceps stretch
92. Alternative hamstring stretch
99. Upper hamstring stretch: lying
103. Calf stretch
105. Combined gastrocnemius/peroneal stretch
106. Achilles and soleus stretch

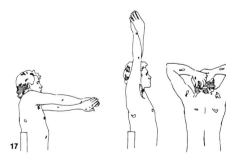
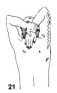

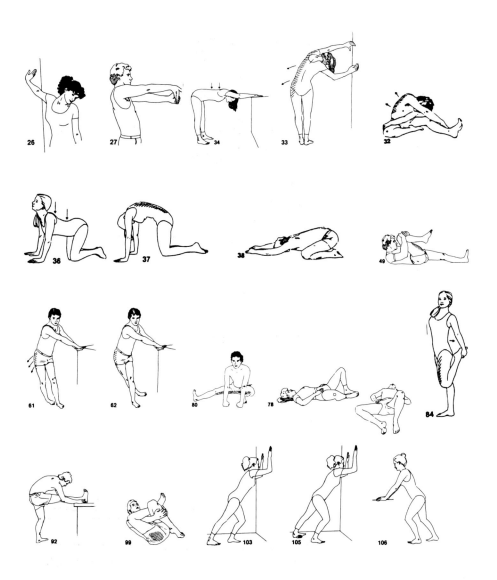

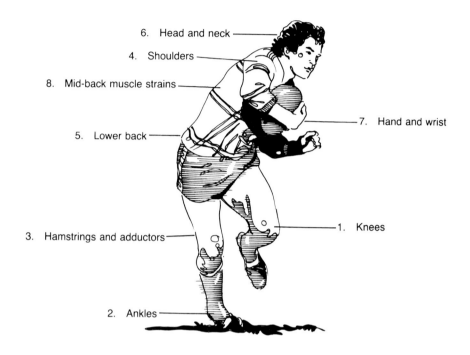

6. Head and neck

4. Shoulders

8. Mid-back muscle strains

7. Hand and wrist

5. Lower back

3. Hamstrings and adductors

1. Knees

2. Ankles

FOOTBALL (RUGBY UNION, RUGBY LEAGUE AND TOUCH)

All codes of football have differing demands. While a good level of general aerobic and anaerobic fitness is essential, players must train specifically for the skills required in their positions.

Because it is a body contact sport, injury in all codes of football is usually due to direct trauma (that is, impact with another player or with the ground). However, unnecessary injury due to inadequate warm-up and preparation too often occurs. Preventative measures are suggested.

Training for these codes of football is quite similar. The key to effective training is not only to establish a base level of fitness but also to practise skills required for the position of play. Both aerobic and anaerobic fitness are essential for a game of rugby.

Training tips

- Adequate pre-season preparation. General cardiovascular fitness should be the priority in the off season and pre-season months, combined with flexibility and strength training. Injury results too often because the player gets too unfit in between seasons.
- Individual player fitness. Each player needs to train to match the specified demands required of his position. General tips for forwards and backs are:
- Forwards need to work on the strength of the upper torso, shoulders, back and especially the neck. Quadriceps, gluteus maximus, calves and hamstrings also need to be strong for the pushing required in scrum work. Commonest injuries for forwards are neck strains, shoulder and lower back problems. Most injuries are of a muscular or ligamentous nature. Overall flexibility balanced by adequate strength training can minimise the risk of injury.

  Additional training should include short distance sprint work and change of direction activities to improve agility, both with and without the ball. Throughout the season, weight training should be continued if possible, but mainly for the neck, shoulders and back. Muscle bulking of the legs should be minimised as this can limit speed, not that long distances at speed are required too often by forwards.
- Agility and speed are foremost for backs. Injuries to backs differ according to the position played but the commonest traumas are hamstring and groin (or adductor) injuries because of the extra kicking required. Major trauma such as knee injuries (common to both forwards and backs) and shoulder strains also occur frequently.

Warm-up

Aerobic classes are an excellent way of warming up for rugby. Flexibility of hamstrings, quadriceps, calves, adductors and lower back should follow a general warm-up. Again this may be incorporated into the warm-up phase of an aerobics or conditioning class or a light jog. Specific warm-up for backs should not just involve static stretching but also dynamic work. This means loosening-up stretches such as high kicks, practising with both legs, gradually increasing the height which the leg goes each time.

This is particularly important for the goal kicker who must also try to keep warm with intermittent stretching throughout the game, even though he may not be directly involved in the game all the time. Change of direction and stop/start running at brief intervals for extended periods of time are essential as part of the warm-up for all backs.

Overall, all positions on field require a high level of stamina, good flexibility, adequate strength, agility skills, co-ordination, good reflexes, ball skills as well as the ability to fall correctly. This latter aspect is often negated in current training programmes. Practice at landing and hitting the ground and passing the ball at the same time is imperative. Avoiding landing on the elbow, or worse still the outstretched hand, can avoid major shoulder ligament damage. The commonest trauma due to this type of body and ground contact is the acromioclavicular joint, which is the bony prominence where the scapula meets the clavicle.

Training should incorporate practice in falling with or without the ball (work with mats can be helpful) and for forwards additional contact work practising scrumming.

Checklist

- If the ground is hard and dry, the falls will also be harder. Let the body roll into its fall where possible. The more relaxed you are when you fall, the less chance of injury. Wet or muddy fields create more sliding injuries. Pay particular attention to hamstrings and adductors to prevent groin injuries.
- Adequate stretching of calves, hamstrings, quadriceps, adductors, lower back, hip flexors, neck and general upper back is needed. Specific warm-up and stretches for forwards and backs should also be done.
- Training of skills specific to position of play need to include:
  — Change of direction activities, including figure eight work
  — Sprint work
  — Ball skills
  — Balance, co-ordination skills with and without the ball, and
  — Agility skills to improve manoeuvrability.
  A further point of interest is that statistics show that most major injuries in these games occur either in the first five minutes of the match or in the third quarter, after the rest at half-time. It seems pre- and mid-match warm-up and stretching would have its benefits.
- Ankle taping can reduce the incidence of sprained ankles. (See Basketball.) If you have knee ligament damage or laxity, a knee guard may provide better support. For corked areas such as the thigh, it is advisable to wear some form of support which keeps the area warm.

Warm-up: Go for a light jog either on the spot or around an oval. Gradually progress to change of direction work such as jogging one way, touching the ground and jogging back the other way in a zig-zag fashion. After stretching all major muscle groups, particularly the lower limb, try to build up the pace and amount of work undertaken while jogging with knees to the chest and so on. Aerobics classes are an ideal way to achieve an effective warm-up and stretch prior to training. Aerobics classes improve flexibility, agility and co-ordination, as well as providing specific stretches for all major muscle groups. PNF stretches are recommended for football.

Football (League, Union and touch) exercise routine

1. Neck flexion
2. Neck extension
3. Neck rotation
4. Neck side flexion
17. Thoracic spine and shoulder mobility exercise
21. Tricep stretch
22. Latissimus dorsi stretch
33. Side trunk stretch
30. Posterior shoulders and thoracic spine stretch: sitting
29. Upper back stretch
26. Wrist, shoulder and neck stretch
80. Adductor stretch: standing/squatting
49. Knee hug stretch
99. Upper hamstring stretch: lying
103. Calf stretch
106. Achilles and soleus stretch
11. Pectoral stretch
61. Hip abductor stretch
62. Advanced hip abductor stretch
84. Quadriceps stretch
85. Quadriceps stretch and hip mobility: lying
86. Hip flexor stretch: kneeling
52. Spinal rotation stretch: sitting
78. Adductor stretch and oblique strengthening

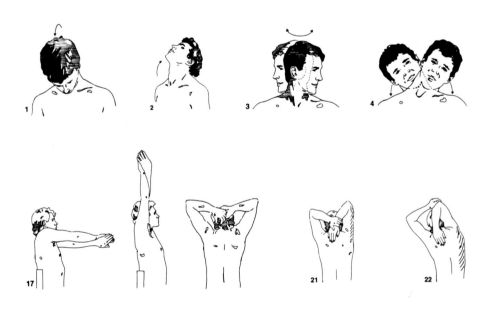

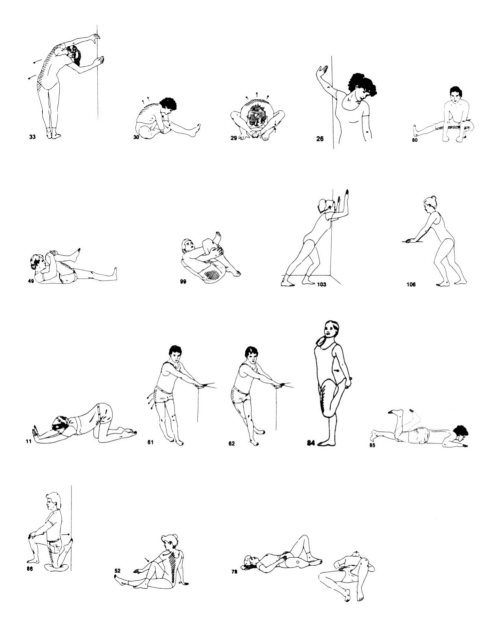

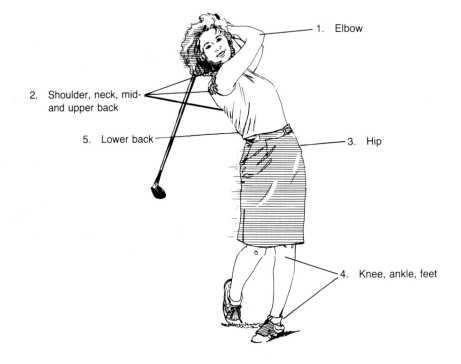

1. Elbow

2. Shoulder, neck, mid-
    and upper back

5. Lower back

3. Hip

4. Knee, ankle, feet

GOLF

While golf does tend to be a very social activity for most, it is not really a very
effective exercise for improving stamina. Even though considerable walking is
involved it is usually not continuous and is usually played at a rather leisurely
pace. However, enjoyment can be greater if warm-up is incorporated into your
golf routine.

Injuries in golf are usually limited to the regions of the elbow, shoulder and
neck, the lower back and to the hip. Inflexibility or poor technique are the usual
reasons why problems occur.

Golfer's elbow

This term refers to pain on the inside or medial aspect of the elbow. It is usually
a tendonitis or bursitis (see Chapter 9) at the origin of the muscle which arises
from the medial epicondyle (the bony prominence on the humerus). It may be
caused by poor technique, muscle imbalance around the shoulder or elbow or
forearm muscles, or it may be due to overtraining. Seek treatment if you experience elbow pain when you play golf. Delay in treatment will mean delay in recovery and return to your sport if rest is prescribed.

Checklist

- Wear supportive golf or walking shoes to ensure you do not trip on the golf course. Be sure to select a size of club suited to the different strokes you need to do.
- Good technique in golf is of prime importance. It is never too late for coaching.
- Walk briskly between holes and continue to do a few stretches throughout your game.
- Combine golf with some form of aerobic activity. Your improved level of fitness will reduce how readily you fatigue when you play and may therefore improve your performance.

Warm-up and cool-down: It is essential to loosen the shoulders and the mid- and lower back prior to play. Large circular swinging movements provide a general warm-up prior to stretching. It is important to simulate the golfing action in your warm-up. Use a golf stick where possible to assist with your stretches, particularly during your warm-up.

Golf exercise routine

  17. Thoracic spine and shoulder mobility exercise
  21. Tricep stretch
  22. Latissimus dorsi stretch
  11. Pectoral stretch
  23. Shoulder rotations: sitting
  24. Shoulder rotations: lying
  28. Thoracic spine and rhomboids stretch
  26. Wrist, shoulder and neck stretch
  18. Thoracic spine and shoulder mobility exercise using a rod. Use the golf club. Do not go all the way behind the back if it is painful.
  30. Posterior shoulders and thoracic spine stretch
  33. Side trunk stretch
  52. Spinal rotation stretch: sitting
  80. Adductor stretch: standing/squatting
  49. Knee hug stretch
117. Ankle mobility
  93. Hamstring stretch: sitting *OR*
  92. Alternative hamstring stretch
  98. Upper hamstring stretch: standing

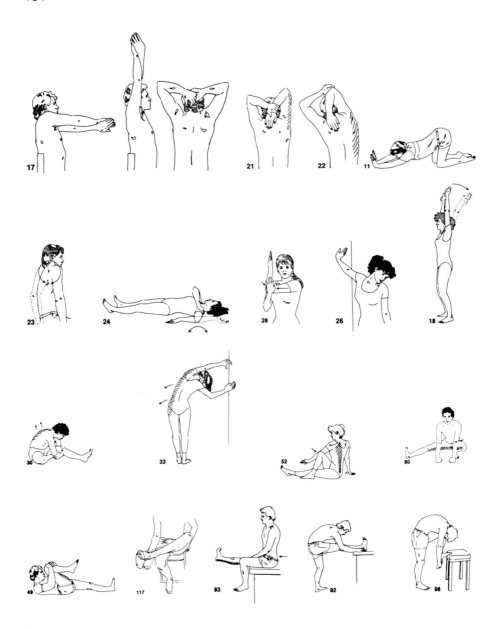

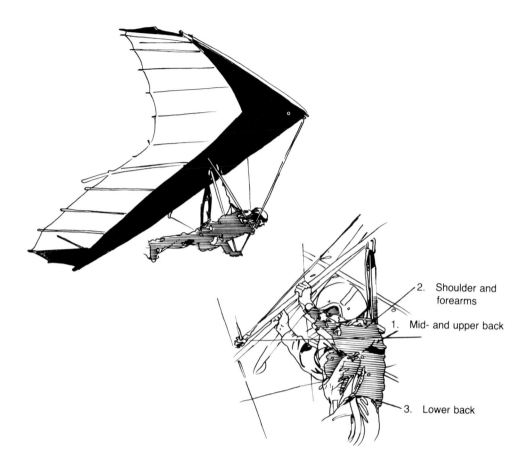

2. Shoulder and
   forearms

1. Mid- and upper back

3. Lower back

HANG-GLIDING

Australia boasts some of the top hang-gliders in the world. While it is a fun
sport, the pleasure and enjoyment can be magnified by taking a few precautions.

Hang-gliding can be very fatiguing, so improved levels of fitness can minimise
this. However, the type of fitness required for hang-gliding is extremely sports
specific. While aerobic fitness does not *directly* influence the glider's ability to
stay in the air, strength and flexibility do.

The demands placed on the upper musculature of the body are enormous. The
lower body pivots around the mid-back (thoracolumbar region) while the
shoulders and mid-back are in a continuous state of interchange between both
isometric (static position of the limbs) and dynamic movement.

Additional strength of the upper back, shoulders and arms can certainly decrease the onset of fatigue while in the air. Not many sports require this type of

continuous strength demand for sometimes up to 3–4 hours.

Combining hang-gliding with sports such as surfboard riding, surf-skiing, swimming or rowing, can assist in maintenance of strength of the musculature of the upper limb. Alternatively, using weight training may be preferred. Unfortunately, this sport is very dependent on the elements, such as the wind and rain, so keeping strength up by simply hang-gliding is usually just not possible.

The main injuries seen from hang-gliding are stiffness in the shoulders and mid-thoracic spine and the upper arms, and often ankle sprains after a poor landing. The risk of major injury in this sport is high if the utmost caution is not taken preparing the apparatus and yourself for the sport.

Checklist

- Obtain specialist help in the maintenance of your equipment. Check for weathered straps, harnesses and so on regularly.
- Be careful loading the glider onto the car, particularly when you are fatigued.
- Include strengthening of the upper torso, abdominals, shoulders, arms, wrists, forearms and back with a regular fitness programme, to enhance your enjoyment of this fun activity and delay the onset of fatigue, particularly after you have finished gliding.

Warm-up: This should include loosening of the shoulders with large movements as well as specific stretches for the shoulders, neck, forearms and back.

Hang-gliding exercise routine

1. Neck flexion
2. Neck extension
3. Neck rotation
4. Neck side flexion
17. Thoracic spine and shoulder mobility exercise
21. Tricep stretch
22. Latissimus dorsi stretch
32. Latissimus dorsi/quadratus lumborum stretch
26. Wrist, shoulder and neck stretch
29. Upper back stretch
34. Advanced thoracic spine mobility
39. Spinal flexion/extension stretch
80. Adductor stretch: standing/squatting
94. Hamstring and lower back stretch
84. Quadriceps stretch
52. Spinal rotation stretch: sitting
98. Upper hamstring stretch
117. Ankle mobility

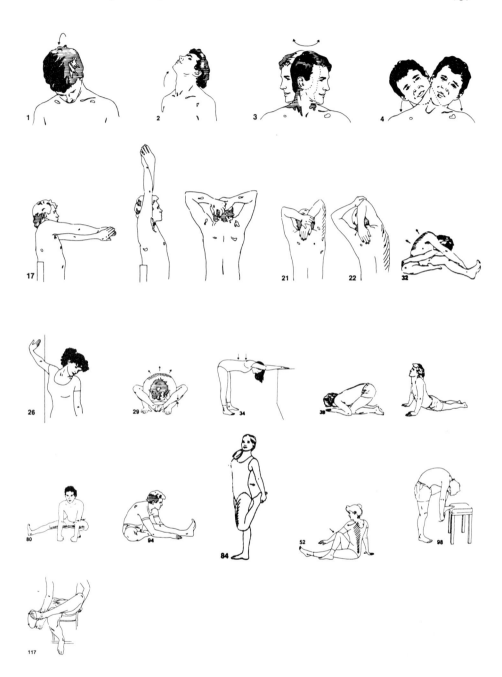

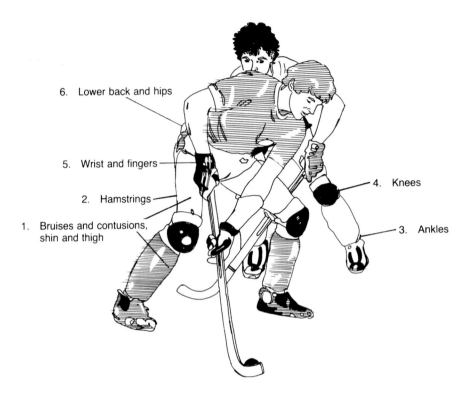

6. Lower back and hips

5. Wrist and fingers

2. Hamstrings

1. Bruises and contusions,
   shin and thigh

4. Knees

3. Ankles

HOCKEY

Hockey is a game requiring a combination of agility, co-ordination, speed of direction and good ball handling skills. All of these are enhanced by improved flexibility, strength and general fitness.

The areas most vulnerable to injury are the lower back and hamstrings, adductors, ankles, knees and hands. Over or inappropriate training can lead to shin soreness and sore lower leg muscles. Bruises and contusions to all parts of the body are also very common.

Though hockey is predominantly an anaerobic form of activity, a base level of aerobic fitness is essential to minimise fatigue during match play. Specific skill training should be practised preferably twice each week between matches, and combined with other forms of fitness. Jogging and aerobics classes are the ideal.

Checklist

- Be sure you have protection for your shins. The goal keeper is advised to wear headgear protection at all times.
- Replace footwear if you are developing blisters too frequently.
- Training specifially for your position of play is critical.
- Attention to ball skills, dribbling (slow and at speed) and attacking must be practised regularly.
- If you are cramping often throughout the game check you are drinking sufficient fluid throughout the game itself as well as prior to your sport.
- Try to combine your hockey training with other sports, particularly aerobic activities.
- Try to keep fit between seasons and particularly pre-season.

Warm-up and cool-down: Adequate warm-up should include a light jog around the oval, followed by stretches to the lower back, hamstrings, calves, adductors, abductors, the shoulders and mid- and upper back. This should be followed by change of direction activities and practice of ball handling skills.

Hockey exercise routine

1. Neck flexion
2. Neck extension
3. Neck rotation
4. Neck side flexion
17. Thoracic spine and shoulder mobility exercise
21. Tricep stretch
22. Latissimus dorsi stretch
26. Wrist, shoulder and neck stretch
32. Latissimus dorsi/quadratus lumborum stretch
33. Side trunk stretch
11. Pectoral stretch
84. Quadriceps stretch
80. Adductor stretch: standing/squatting
61. Hip abductor stretch
94. Hamstring and lower back stretch
78. Adductor stretch and oblique strengthening
103. Calf stretch
105. Combined gastrocnemius/peroneal stretch
106. Achilles and soleus stretch
117. Ankle mobility

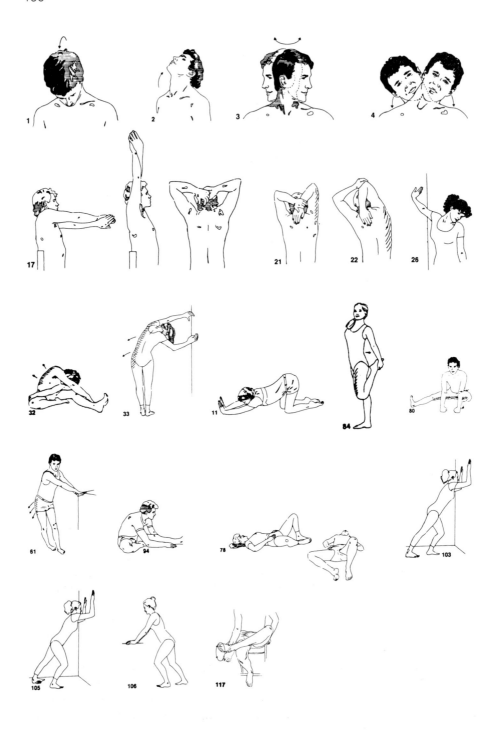

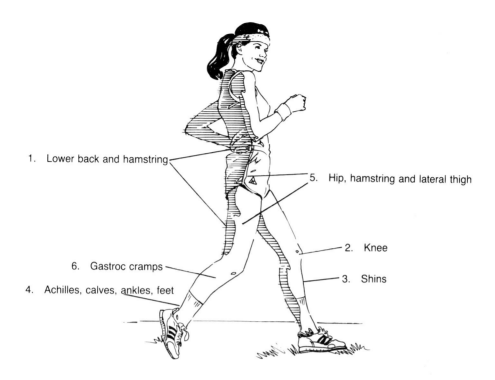

1. Lower back and hamstring

5. Hip, hamstring and lateral thigh

2. Knee

6. Gastroc cramps

3. Shins

4. Achilles, calves, ankles, feet

JOGGING/RUNNING

Jogging continues to be a popular activity for many. By itself, it is an ideal activity for keeping aerobically fit, but it is also an excellent means of keeping fit for other activities. The words 'jogging' and 'running' are used interchangeably in this text.

The main problem area for runners is usually the lower limb. Foot and achilles problems, knee pain, tightness of the hamstring and lower back and sciatica are the most commonly occurring jogger complaints.

When we consider that we put seven to nine times our own body weight through each leg when we are running, and that we do this many times throughout our jog, it becomes fairly clear why any slight problem will become magnified by this form of activity. The main reasons why injuries occur and a simple solution are shown below.

INJURY CAUSE	INJURY PREVENTION
1. Skeletal, bowed legs, femur or tibia etc.	Get a postural and skeletal assessment
2. Foot problems (usually overpronation)	Corrective orthotics (prescribed by a podiatrist)
3. Muscle/tendon inflexibility	Regular stretching daily, prior to and at the completion of your run
4. Muscle/tendon strength imbalance	Identifying weakness, stretching these muscles/tendons and assessing your own posture will assist this
5. Running on hard or uneven surfaces	Run on softer or a variety of surfaces. Do not run in one direction all the time
6. Inferior running shoes	Buy quality brand running shoes suitable for your foot type
7. Poor running style	Usually related to muscle imbalance or inflexibility but you may need to learn how to run; relaxing as you run is a key factor to good style. Do not run on the toes, but maintain a comfortable almost flat-footed gait. Let one leg 'fall' in front of the other as you jog.
8. Stress and overtraining	Reduce the intensity of your programme; rest and review your jogging programme; remember three times per week of 20–30 minutes of aerobic exercise is the minimum required to keep the heart and lungs fit

Commonly asked questions

Why is pronation often stated as the cause of so many joggers' problems?

Pronation has been blamed for everything from knee and back pain to headaches. While there may be truth in some of these cases, pronation is generally far too often blamed for problems caused by other factors which may be treatable. The first point to note is that pronation is a normal part of the gait cycle. When we walk, each foot spends time on the ground called the 'stance' phase and in the air, this is the 'swing' phase. The stance phase comprises up to 80 per cent of the gait cycle and the swing phase comprises the rest.

During stance, whether it be in walking or jogging, the heel strikes the ground first, then the foot rolls inwards letting the arch of the foot collapse. This is called pronation. Next the foot, in sequence with the external rotators of the hip, rolls upward and out. This is called supination. The foot then returns to a 'neutral' position where a slight rolling in and out at the base of the toes occurs prior to push-off. The final push-off should occur between the base of the big toe and the second toe.

Therefore, pronation is a normal phase of any walking or jogging motion. However, weak ankles, tight calves, weak hip external rotators or lower back muscles, tight adductors, weak foot intrinsic musculature can all contribute to excessive pronation occurring. Whether the above structures create the over-pronation or whether the foot itself through age, musculoskeletal imbalances, heredity factors, or lifestyle habits is pronated, is not definitive.

What is clear is that while orthotics may correct the overpronation, if these other factors noted above are not attended to, the problem may recur.

Will the arch supports I can get from a chemist assist with feet problems?

No, these arch supports are not individually tailored and custom made for your foot. You need to have an average foot and usually have a choice of only one of three sizes! Alternatively, a podiatrist will make a cast of your foot and mould an 'orthotic' and reinforce it to suit your needs. You must keep regular check-ups with your podiatrist however as your needs may change as you wear your orthotics in.

However, the mass-produced arch supports bought from chemists are suitable for some people. If you are not engaged in regular exercise they may be sufficient for providing extra support for the foot. Most female, and often male, dress shoe designs do not provide any support for the arch of the foot so these non-custom made supports are certainly better than no support, particularly if your job requires long hours standing on your feet and you currently find your legs and feet are tired after each day.

Similarly, for the older age group, these arch supports inside their shoes can assist with fallen arches and promote more efficient circulation through the legs, particularly if regular walking is performed as exercise. If pain commences when you wear these supports then do not continue wearing them. Seek advice from a podiatrist to find what is suitable for you.

Do inner soles with no arch support, but which are claimed to decrease the shock that goes through my body when I jog, really work?

Scientific tests have certainly shown these products (sold under a variety of brand names) dissipate the force of shock when this is applied to them. However, the recovery time for the shock absorbing qualities to return to the substance used for the inner sole, is often greater than the time taken before the foot is placed down again — particularly in jogging. This means the shock absorption is markedly reduced. People who do seem to gain benefits from these supports are again the older age group who get sore feet or aching knees or back after sport, particularly tennis, netball or golf. The other limiting factor of these supports is that they are very heavy so quite unsuited for distance runners and joggers. Nevertheless, if you find they help a persistent problem you have been suffering from, wear them as they can do little, if no, harm.

How do I know which jogging shoe is right for me?

There are so many jogging shoes on the market today it is certainly difficult to know which one is right for you. Most brands provide the basic features required for jogging, therefore it is totally unwise to be in a regular running programme using tennis or basketball shoes since these are not designed with the appropriate features to protect one from injuries.

Modern running shoes are designed to reduce impact loading and control excessive foot motion. Both these factors help prevent the onset of injury. Other important features to look for when purchasing a running shoe are:

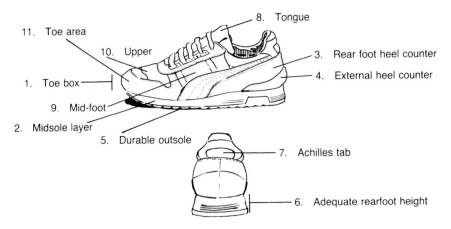

8.3   Key features of a jogging shoe

The heel counter on a tennis or netball shoe does not have the wide base that the jogging shoe does.

- Comfortable fit, this includes allowing a little extra length for foot slide and the increase in foot size which can occur during running.
- A stable rear foot heel counter to control excessive pronation.
- Adequate heel raise (12 – 15 millimetres) for protection of the calf and achilles tendon.
- Adequate absorption in the rear and forefoot as these are the areas which absorb the impact loading the most.
- A roomy section to prevent bruised toenails.
- A flexible midsole.

The pattern of shoe wear on the old shoes will be a good guide when selecting the next pair of running shoes. Old shoes can often give hints as to problems with the running style. If shoe shape is excessively distorted, it usually means a shoe with increased motion control in the rear foot is needed. Figure 8.3 shows the key features one needs to look at when choosing a shoe. Remember, if the shoe is uncomfortable when you put it on in the shop, this will be magnified when you run. Try to give a short test run on the shoes before buying them. Do not just sit down when trying them on.

1. *Toe box:* Adequate height/length to prevent blisters and bruised toenails.
2. *Midsole:* Important shock absorbing layer.
3. *Rear foot heel counter:* Firm moulded plastic; stabilises heel and rear foot in shoe.
4. *External heel counter:* Additional feature to aid in pronation control.
5. *Durable outsole:* Important for surface traction and durability.
6. *Adequate rear foot height:* To relieve stress of achilles and calf muscle group.
7. *Achilles tab:* Used to help pull shoe on (often misnamed as achilles protector).
8. *Tongue:* Well padded to protect foot from lacing pressure. (Pain on the top of the foot can be due to tight lacing.)
9. *Mid-foot:* Reinforced to add stability to mid-foot zone.
10. *Upper:* Usually mesh or nylon for lightweight permeability.
11. *Toe area:* Reinforced to preserve shoe shape and add forefoot support.

Why do so many joggers get back pain often called sciatica?

The previous questions indicated how much load is taken through the body when we jog. Therefore any imbalance in the lower limb may result in back pain. The commonest type of back complaint from joggers is usually musculoligamentous. Factors such as tight hamstring, calf and lower back muscles, inadequate footwear, inappropriate training regime, and running with an injury forcing the body to compensate, are the more common reasons for onset of backache.

Sciatica is the term used to refer to pain associated with impingement of the sciatic nerve. This may occur due to all the above reasons, but it often originates from some type of joint problem occurring at the junction of L5 S1. This is the junction of the lowest lumbar vertebra and the level of the sacrum. While all the lumbar vertebrae move, the five sacral ones do not, which creates a lot of load being taken through this joint, because of the repetitive jarring that occurs in jogging. Muscle spasms of the lower back and hip extensors can place strain and pressure on underlying structures such as the sciatic nerve.

Pain radiating to the buttock or down one leg is commonly associated with sciatic pain. Treatment is essential to ease the problem and to identify why it occurred in the first place and what measures can be taken to prevent it recurring. Doing the exercises for back care in Chapter 7 will ease mild cases of sciatica.

Checklist

• Ensure you have adequate and appropriate footwear. Do your shoes need replacing? Do you wear your shoes down unevenly or wear through the top of your shoe? If so, it may be because you are running in the one direction all the time or running on uneven camber.

- Do you have leg length difference or a foot problem? Consult a sports specialist or podiatrist if you think you do.
- Are you stretching daily? Do you take a rest day, or at least do another form of physical activity (such as swimming) each week?
- Do not neglect stretching of the shoulders and upper limb. Stiffness between the scapulae is common in joggers. Relax your shoulders when you run.
- Perform regular strengthening exercises, particularly if you have a sedentary occupation.
- Make sure you rest when you are injured. If you do not, other areas of your body will compensate and the time of rest when you are eventually forced out of action by your injury will be greatly increased.
- Are you wearing the appropriate clothing for cold and warm weather?
- Do you feel relaxed when you run? Do you have good style and technique? If not, you may need a postural or musculoskeletal assessment. Do you over-pronate? Are you tired all the time when you jog? If so, you may be over-training.

Warm-up and cool-down: Loosen up the arms and shoulders and do a few minutes' brisk walking, just to get the circulation going prior to stretching. Pay particular attention to lower limb muscles. Most of the emphasis of your stretching will be during cool-down once you have gone for your run, and are a bit warmer.

Jogging exercise routine

103. Calf stretch
106. Achilles and soleus stretch
105. Combined gastrocnemius/peroneal stretch
 84. Quadriceps stretch
 85. Quadriceps stretch and hip mobility: lying
 97. Combined hamstring and adductor stretch
 98. Upper hamstring stretch *OR*
 99. Upper hamstring stretch: lying
 23. Shoulder rotations: sitting
 29. Upper back stretch
 34. Advanced thoracic spine mobility
 17. Thoracic spine and shoulder mobility exercise
 50. Spinal rotation stretch: lying
 61. Hip abductor stretch
 78. Adductor stretch and oblique strengthening
 64. Lateral rotators of the hip strengthening
 94. Hamstring and lower back stretch
 49. Knee hug stretch
 48. Pelvis and lower back release
111. Shin strengthening
  6. Wall exercise

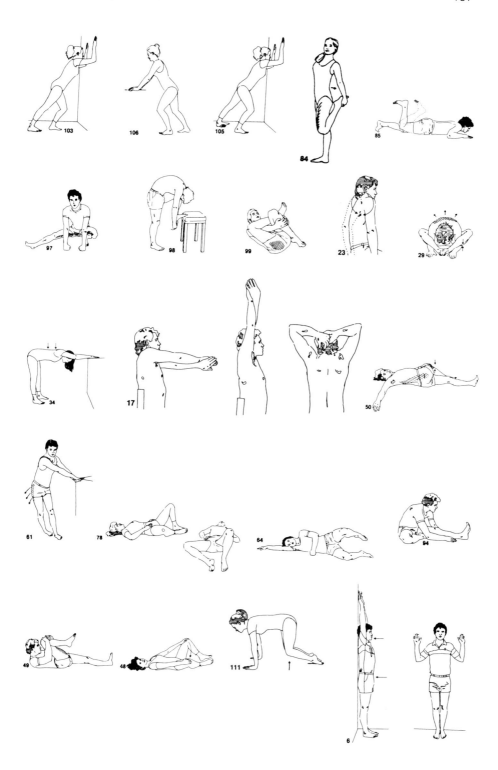

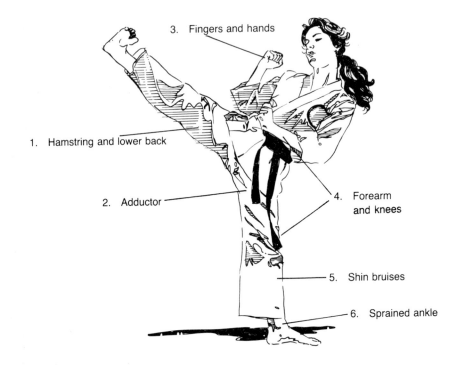

3. Fingers and hands

1. Hamstring and lower back

2. Adductor

4. Forearm and knees

5. Shin bruises

6. Sprained ankle

MARTIAL ARTS

There are many forms of martial arts, each requiring slightly different skills. All forms require strength, flexibility, co-ordination, speed, control, agility and mental discipline to execute a specified movement. Some forms of martial arts incorporate grappling styles, others have more striking movements. In the latter, some incorporate softer movements such as Tai Chi and Pa Kua while others involve more aggressive moves such as Tae Kwan Do and Karate.

The most common injuries are muscle strains of the adductors, hamstrings, shoulder and lower back. Styles featuring more spinning actions (Tae Kwan Do) can cause hip flexor and external oblique strain. Ankle sprains do happen, though these are less common. Contusions and bruises also occur frequently due to sparring, both on the forearms, which block a kick, and on the shins.

Beginners are certainly the most vulnerable to injury, particularly their hands and fingers. The usual reasons for this are, firstly, they do not keep their fists closed when sparring and when they 'miss-hit' a forearm block, and secondly because they practise a style which encourages open hands (such as Kung Fu). While still learning, beginners do not often practise sparring frequently enough and the co-ordination in blocking is therefore lacking. This subsequently leads to injury. Beginners should never go to a class which is too advanced for them.

In some forms of martial arts, stone bruises of the heel may happen. This is usually from hard and/or repeated landings or contact from flying kick practice. Early signs of this form of injury should be attended to as they are very slow to heal. The main consideration for preventing injury in all forms of martial arts is technique. Each style adopts a slightly different method for kicking, particularly with respect to the back. Tae Kwan Do, for instance, uses a much straighter hip/back alignment than other styles. A combination of strength and flexibility of both the back and the hips is essential for all styles.

Another mechanism of injury is if a limb is not tensed strongly just before impact. This protects the knees (and the elbows) from hyperextension or contacting at an awkward angle on impact. This is often not taught to beginners. Regular practice of 'air-kicks', in addition to work with heavy targets, is essential to develop firm focus at the end of range of a kick. This minimises the risk of hyperextension.

Will knuckle and chop work cause arthritis in later years?

This is a very common question asked by students. Martial arts experts claim it need not, at least no more than any other sport, if some basic precautions are taken. This type of work should be progressed very slowly, over 2 to 3 years at least. Any hand injury (particularly the knuckle) should have no work on it till it is 100 per cent recovered. Similarly, no breaking should be done until the knuckle has been correctly 'toughened' for at least 2 years. Many instructors teach their students to break after a few months. There is a risk of injury if this is done, however. It is preferable to do knuckle work on a surface with some give, such as wood, and to begin hitting softly. The technique should involve pressing through a target after the strike, as opposed to bouncing off the surface.

Checklist

- Be sure that mats are safely lying down to prevent risk of tripping, if they are being used.
- Repetition for enhancement of a skill must not be practised at the expense of the body which may be overloaded causing fatigue and poor form with possible injury resulting.
- Good form when executing kicks or arm punches can minimise unnecessary load on a joint, particularly the knees, wrist and knuckles, the shoulder and the back. Depending on which form of martial arts you do, weight training may provide you with added strength. Light weights, not heavy poundage, is to be recommended.

Warm-up: Must include both full range activities for the arms and legs prior to fast speed kicks. Pace of the warm-up should be increased gradually. Stretches for all parts of the body are essential.

P.N.F. stretching is ideal for this sport. Hamstrings, adductors, lower back, knees, ankles and shoulders must all be stretched well.

Martial arts exercise routine

1. Neck flexion
2. Neck extension
3. Neck rotation

  4. Neck side flexion
11. Pectoral stretch
17. Thoracic spine and shoulder mobility exercise
18. Thoracic spine and shoulder mobility exercise using a rod
34. Advanced thoracic spine mobility
33. Side trunk stretch
32. Latissimus dorsi/quadratus lumborum stretch
41. Lower back stretch
42. Advanced lower back stretch
43. Advanced lower back stretch with hip rotation
80. Adductor stretch: standing/squatting
78. Adductor stretch and oblique strengthening
50. Spinal rotation stretch: lying *OR* 51. Double leg spinal rotation
84. Quadriceps stretch
103. Calf stretch
106. Achilles and soleus stretch

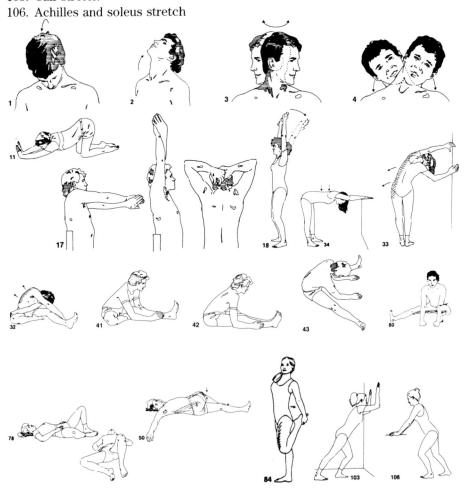

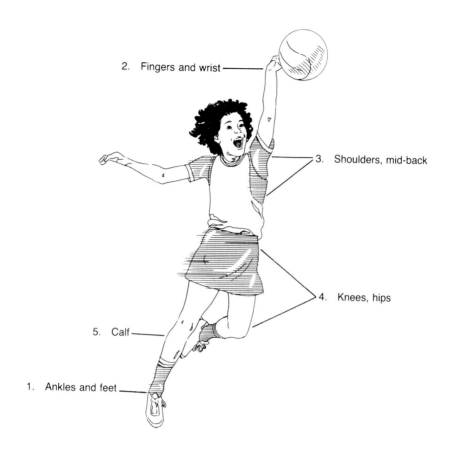

2. Fingers and wrist

3. Shoulders, mid-back

4. Knees, hips

5. Calf

1. Ankles and feet

NETBALL

In Australia, more women play this sport than any other. Men's netball has become popular more recently. The highest incidence of injury is sprained ankles, finger and wrist trauma, while knee, shoulder, neck or back injuries are less frequent.

In theory, netball is a non-contact sport, but in practice, once a team of seven players starts moving around within a limited space and starts trying to win and outdo its opposition, contact is invariably bound to happen — whether on purpose or accidentally. Many of the traumas to the hands, though, do occur when the ball is caught at an awkward angle. If damage to the fingers and hand is only minor, taping the sprained finger to its neighbour (Figure 8.4) can assist while playing. If ice does not ease the pain within 24 hours, consult a therapist for treatment.

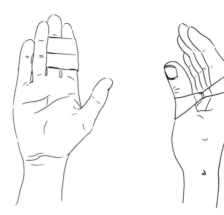

8.4   Variations of finger taping

Netball shoes

Netball shoes, designed for agility, are preferable to the higher basketball boot. If you tend to have weak ankles with overstretched ligaments, try taping first (see Basketball) and if this does not work then try the higher boot. Some agility is lost but it does tend to be a personal choice. Basketball tends to attract taller and larger framed individuals than netball. This means that additional stability of the lower extremity is preferable for the high speed changes of direction required. The height of netballers tends to be less and the speed of the game not as great (though not always) as basketball.

Checklist

- If playing on hard surfaces, try to mix your training between softer and harder surfaces so that you do not develop problems such as shin splints.
- Tape fingers or the ankle preventatively if you sustain sprains to these areas frequently.
- Combine your netball with other forms of aerobic or anaerobic activity.
- Try to train between matches to improve your agility, co-ordination and ball handling skills.
- A basic level of aerobic fitness combined with anaerobic fitness is essential for netball. Practice of agility skills, shuttle sprints and ball handling skills will sharpen your reflexes in a game.

Warm-up: A light jog around the court, followed by stretches to the hamstrings, adductors, calves, lower back, shoulders and wrists should precede practice of ball skills and agility skills. Shuttle sprints on the court should be incorporated in warm-up.

Netball exercise routine

  1. Neck flexion
  2. Neck extension
  3. Neck rotation
  4. Neck side flexion
 17. Thoracic spine and shoulder mobility exercise
 27. Wrist and finger stretch
 21. Tricep stretch
 22. Latissimus dorsi stretch
 33. Side trunk stretch
 28. Thoracic spine and rhomboids stretch
 29. Upper back stretch
 41. Lower back stretch
 34. Advanced thoracic spine mobility
 31. Posterior shoulder and thoracic spine stretch
 80. Adductor stretch: standing/squatting
 52. Spinal rotation stretch: sitting
 84. Quadriceps stretch
 91. Hamstring stretch
 49. Knee hug stretch
103. Calf stretch
106. Achilles and soleus stretch
117. Ankle mobility

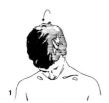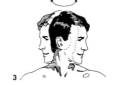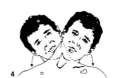

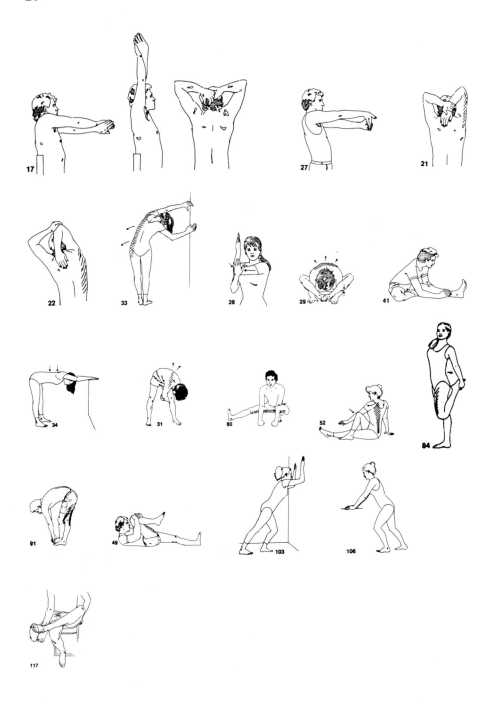

2. Mid- and upper back

4. Shoulder

3. Forearm and wrist

1. Lower back

ROWING, KAYAKING, CANOEING AND SURF-SKI RIDING

While each of these sports differs from each other, the functional demands placed on the individual playing them is similar. Whether for leisure, pleasure or competitive reasons the enjoyment of each of these activities can be enhanced by additional fitness and appropriate stretching.

The main problem areas for all these sports are the lower back, shoulders, forearms, and a sore coccyx and buttocks in kayaking.

The major reasons rowers develop back problems are because of an inadequate warm-up and preparation, and usually muscle imbalance.

Rowers tend to train early each morning and, therefore, the lack of incentives to warm-up at this time of day is often understandable! However, jumping out of bed and heading straight off to lift the boats out of storage, followed by a heavy training session, is very demanding on even the fittest body. A general loosening up of both the upper and lower body, as well as the torso, can not only prevent post-exercise soreness but also minimise lower back strain.

One of the other problems for many rowers, predisposing them to back problems, is muscle imbalance. It is imperative to try and row on both sides of the boat. This is particularly important in training for the teenager who takes up rowing, where imbalance can be difficult to reverse in later years. Also, it is very easy to row using the more flexible thoracic spine (stretching forward from the upper and mid-back), rather than using the power gained from using the quadriceps, hip and lower back. Placing strips of sports tape from the clavicle to the opposite side on the thoracic spine, on both shoulders to pull the shoulders back can assist with teaching correct rowing technique, if an individual is pulling from an already flexible upper spine. Consult a physiotherapist who performs taping for postural correction if you are unsure how to use this method yourself. (See Chapter 3.)

Preparation in between training sessions is also imperative for even the 'social' rower. A general stretching and strengthening programme for the entire body, not just the upper limb, will ensure a balance of muscle strength is retained, reducing the risk of musculoskeletal trauma.

Weight training is an ideal adjunct to rowing and can assist with detecting muscle imbalances as well as providing more strength when competing.

Checklist

- Pay more attention to warm-up on cold mornings. Be sure your surfski or kayak is not too small for you. This places added stress on your lumbar spine.
- Balance (particularly for kayaking, canoeing and surf-skiing) should be developed, and tipping in still water before you practise in 'white water' is critical.
- If kayaking, try to keep shifting the buttocks a little from side to side, to prevent numbness in the legs occurring due to compression on the sciatic nerve.
- Try to practise rowing on both sides in training.
- Try to balance your rowing with other forms of activities to improve your general aerobic fitness level. Weight training and regular stretching are ideal.

Warm-up: Loosen the shoulders with large circular movements, forwards and backwards. If training in summer go for a quick swim before you get in the boat. If not, adequately stretch all major muscle groups, with particular attention to the shoulders, mid- and upper back, the lower back, the hip flexors, adductors, and hamstrings.

Rowing exercise routine

   1. Neck flexion
   2. Neck extension
   3. Neck rotation
   4. Neck side flexion
  33. Side trunk stretch
  22. Latissimus dorsi stretch
  21. Tricep stretch
  84. Quadriceps stretch
  28. Thoracic spine and rhomboids stretch
  17. Thoracic spine and shoulder mobility exercise
  29. Upper back stretch
  31. Upper back and posterior shoulder stretch: standing
  80. Adductor stretch: standing/squatting
  34. Advanced thoracic spine mobility
  11. Pectoral stretch
  40. Passive back extension stretch
  94. Hamstring and lower back stretch
  50. Spinal rotation stretch: lying
  73. Beginners' lower abdominals strengthening
  74. Intermediate lower abdominals strengthening
  49. Knee hug stretch
  38. Lower back release

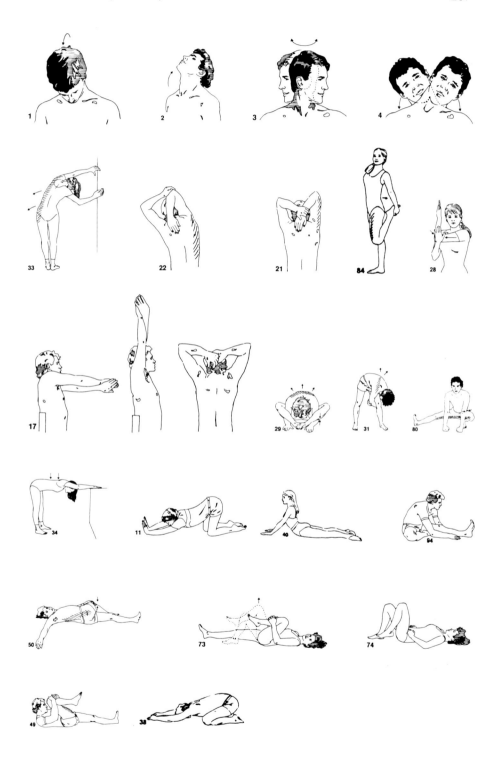

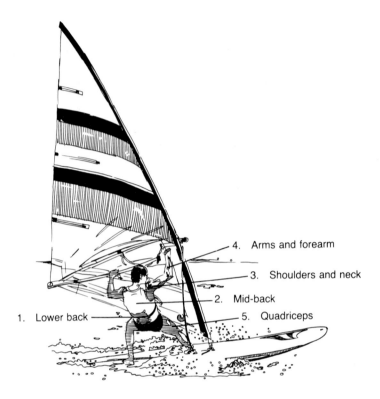

4. Arms and forearm

3. Shoulders and neck

2. Mid-back

1. Lower back

5. Quadriceps

SAILBOARDING (WINDSURFING)

This sport has increased markedly in popularity during the past 5 or 6 years. Because of the fun nature of the sport major injuries are minimal. However, post-exercise soreness can be prevented with adequate warm-up stretching.

Using a sailboard or learning to windsurf can be a tedious, and sometimes even a painful, experience! Like any sport, the key to learning is patience, practice and developing good technique. One of the biggest mistakes beginners make is when they are pulling the sail out of the water. Instead of using their legs and thighs they use their arms and back and usually stick their buttocks out as the sail comes up. This invariably leads to muscle fatigue, which impedes developing good technique, and post-exercise soreness (usually of the lower back or of the arms) occurs.

Be sure to get advice from a skilled rider to improve your technique.

Like any sport the ultimate goal is to permit the body to be as relaxed as possible to achieve optimum effectiveness from our muscles. Have you noticed how relaxed an experienced sailboard rider looks even though he or she may be moving at high speeds? Good technique is the key to mastering this fun sport.

Checklist

- Wear a wet suit in cold weather or cold water, to prevent cramping or unnecessary strain or fatigue of the muscles.
- Check the height of the cross-bar. It should be approximately shoulder height. It is inefficient to have it higher.
- Try to use a harness to lessen the work on the arms where possible.
- Loosen up and warm-up well prior to sailboarding and stretch the evening after you have windsurfed. This will prevent post-exercise soreness, particularly if you are learning.

Warm-up: Ideally a light jog along the water's edge will loosen the body up, or alternatively, having a quick swim. Stretches of the shoulders, triceps, upper and lower back, hip flexors, thigh and calves both before and after sailboarding will enhance your enjoyment of this sport.

Sailboarding exercise routine

22. Latissimus dorsi stretch
21. Tricep stretch
28. Thoracic spine and rhomboids stretch
23. Shoulder rotations: sitting
24. Shoulder rotations: lying
17. Thoracic spine and shoulder mobility exercise
52. Spinal rotation stretch: sitting
98. Upper hamstring stretch: standing
33. Side trunk stretch
91. Hamstring stretch: standing
49. Knee hug stretch
84. Quadriceps stretch
80. Adductor stretch: standing/squatting
103. Calf stretch
106. Achilles and soleus stretch

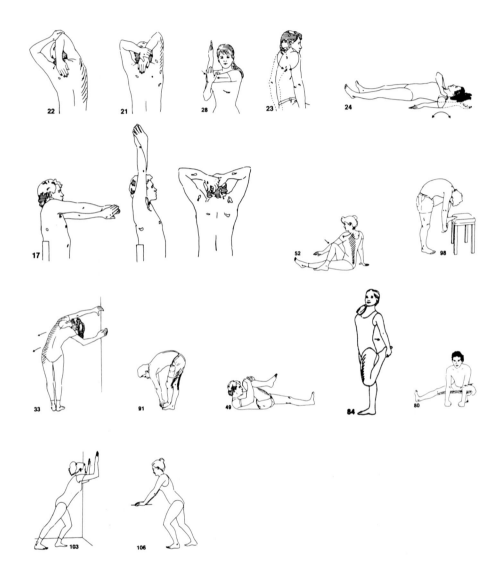

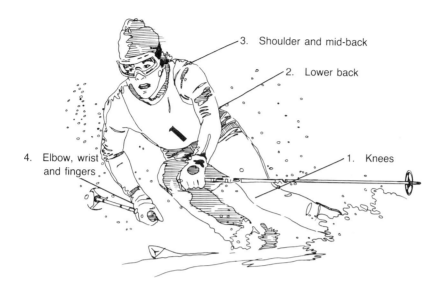

3. Shoulder and mid-back

2. Lower back

4. Elbow, wrist
    and fingers

1. Knees

SNOW-SKIING

Downhill skiing

This fun activity can not only be hazardous but frustrating if sore muscles result each time one skis. Unfortunately, it is against all our better instincts to lean forward when we are learning, so muscle bruises and minor strains are many. Unfortunately the better the skier often the higher the speeds achieved. Therefore, the worse the injury if a fall occurs. Knees and shoulders are the commonest sites of injury in skiing.

While it may seem inappropriate, it is still very important to warm-up before catching a lift up the slopes. When our muscles are stiff and tight we are much more vulnerable to unjury when we fall than if we are stretched out and loosened up. The ideal is to try and do a general warm-up *prior* to going out on the slopes. Loosen up the shoulders with large swinging movements, then lie on your back and do leg cycling, bringing the opposite elbow to each knee. This will loosen the legs and the hips. Next loosen the ankles and knees with circular movements (simulate the skiing action). Now you are ready to do your stretching. Particularly focus on the hamstrings, adductors, quadriceps, hip flexors, shoulders and back.

Cross-country skiing

The demands placed on the body of the cross-country skier differ slightly from those of the downhiller. The work is physically more demanding and mastering good technique can prevent many potential problems occurring. Anterior hip pain, thigh soreness, back and shoulder stiffness are the commonest problem areas. Cross-country skiers usually have very strong and balanced muscles, but being unfit can lead readily to fatigue.

Cross-country skiing is a little like ice skating. Each foot should glide ahead of the other. Beginners often make hard work of it because they try to push each leg in front of the other. Thinking of transferring weight from one leg to the other can assist with refining technique. Because of the greater dynamic muscle action required in this sport, the thighs and hip flexors can get very tight. If you take a break after you have skied for a few hours try to stretch these a little before continuing on. The distance covered by cross-country skiers is often greater than downhillers so muscles are used for longer periods of time. Therefore, fatigue may be greater. Stretching after a day's skiing, therefore, will minimise muscle soreness and tightness the next day.

Checklist

- Do not head for the steepest slopes or the highest moguls on your first run of the day. Work up to these by skiing the less challenging slopes first.
- Boots should not be too tight nor too loose. Try to get a ski expert to assist you with fitting the right size.
- Bindings should be secure and firm but still able to release readily when you fall.
- Do not ski at out-of-control speeds. This is when collisions and major injuries occur. Use common sense on the slopes at all times to minimise risk of injury both to yourself and to others.
- If you get unusual knee, foot or hip pain when you ski you may need orthotics in your shoes. Consult a sports specialist pre-season.
- Pre-season fitness training is essential to maximise your enjoyment while skiing. Aerobics and jogging are ideal ways to improve and maintain your general level of fitness, if you are only skiing on weekends.

Snow-skiing exercise routine

  22. Latissimus dorsi stretch
  21. Tricep stretch
  17. Thoracic spine and shoulder mobility exercise
  31. Upper back and posterior shoulder stretch: standing
  34. Advanced thoracic spine mobility
  98. Upper hamstring stretch: standing
  80. Adductor stretch: standing/squatting
  84. Quadriceps stretch
103. Calf stretch
106. Achilles and soleus stretch
  32. Latissimus dorsi/quadratus lumborum stretch
  33. Side trunk stretch
  11. Pectoral stretch
  52. Spinal rotation stretch: sitting
  38. Lower back release

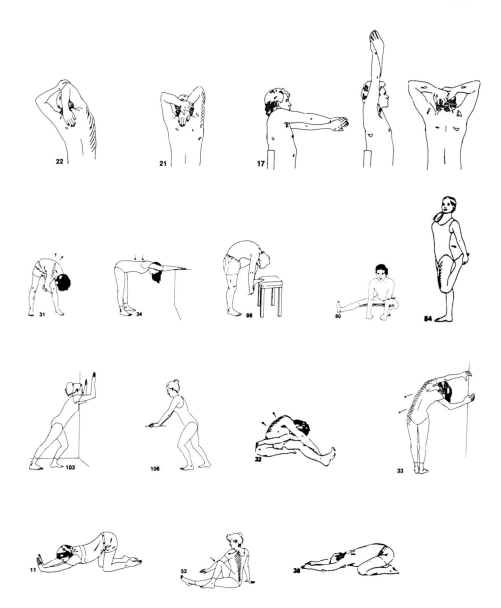

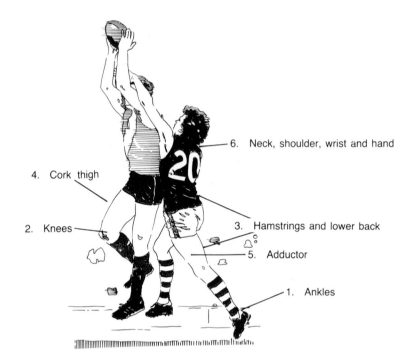

6. Neck, shoulder, wrist and hand

4. Cork thigh

2. Knees

3. Hamstrings and lower back

5. Adductor

1. Ankles

SOCCER/AUSTRALIAN FOOTBALL

General principles of training for Australian football (VFL) and soccer players are similar to those outlined in the section on football. These include general aerobic fitness, flexibility, co-ordination, strength, agility skills and ball control work.

The main differences in soccer and Australian football to other codes though is the greater degree of agility required by all players and the extra balance and co-ordination required by the ankles, knees and hips to manoeuvre the ball. Lack of flexibility of the lower limb or inadequate stretching or warm-up can quickly lead to unnecessary injury.

Soccer and Australian football players also cover greater distances of the field throughout their game so training needs to meet this demand. There is also a lot more jumping and running backwards over longer distances than in other codes of football. This should be practised specifically in training.

The type of injuries seen in soccer and Australian football are indicative of their slightly different stresses. The commonest injuries seen in these sports are groin injuries (adductor strains), hamstring strains, ankle and knee ligament sprains, and minor traumas to fingers and major trauma such as concussion.

Checklist

• Take extra precautions on a wet day when the field is muddy. The more re-

laxed you are when you fall the less prone you are to injury. The same principle applies on a hard, dry field.
- Taping of ankles and knees (see Basketball) can reduce the risk of injury.
- Each player should focus on the demands required in his position of play.
- Specificity of training for these types of football can reduce onset of fatigue in
  match play. A basic level of aerobic fitness needs to be combined with anaerobic work. Shuttle sprints, change of direction work, and running backwards
  at varying speeds, combined with ball handling skills, jumping, goal kicking,
  and so on, should be an integral part of training.

Warm-up: A general warm-up utilising all major muscle groups is essential.
An aerobics class is excellent for all-round conditioning fitness, combining
stretching, strengthening, agility and co-ordination skills. Failing this, a light jog
followed by stretching, and slowly increasing the pace of the running, is ideal.
Backwards, forwards, sideways movements and figure eight pattern work to
improve agility should precede both training and match games.

Stretches for all players should include static and dynamic stretching, and
whenever possible, partner stretching using PNF principles.

Soccer/Australian football exercise routine

1. Neck flexion
2. Neck extension
3. Neck rotation
4. Neck side flexion
21. Tricep stretch
17. Thoracic spine and shoulder mobility exercise
29. Upper back stretch
11. Pectoral stretch
32. Latissimus dorsi/quadratus lumborum stretch
33. Side trunk stretch
12. Pectoral and tricep strengthening
13. Shoulder girdle strengthening
14. Full push-up
60. Advanced hip stretch
40. Passive back extension stretch
49. Knee hug stretch
93. Hamstring stretch: sitting
64. Lateral rotators strengthening
80. Adductor stretch: standing/squatting
81. Adductor stretch: sitting
84. Quadriceps stretch
103. Calf stretch
106. Achilles and soleus stretch
117. Ankle mobility

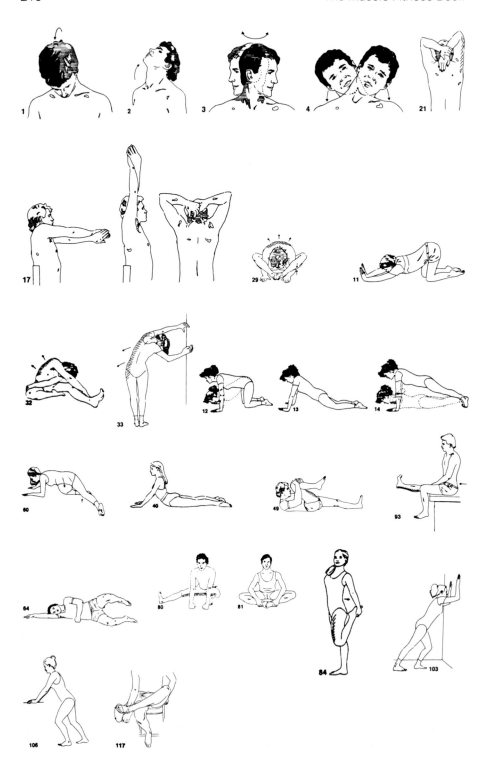

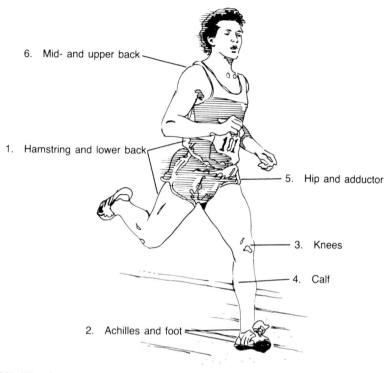

6. Mid- and upper back

1. Hamstring and lower back

5. Hip and adductor

3. Knees

4. Calf

2. Achilles and foot

SPRINTING

The main difference between joggers and sprinters is obviously pace. Also, sprinting is almost a solely anaerobic activity while jogging is usually aerobic. Apart from athletes who sprint competitively, most individuals who incorporate sprinting as part of their fitness regime do so to assist with speed in their particular sport. If you are quite content with your jogging programme then sprinting is not necessarily suitable for you. However, if you are trying to decrease your times in your fun runs then sprinting is an ideal way to achieve this.

The main biomechanical aspect that differs between jogging and sprinting is that sprinters spend most of their time on their forefeet and on their toes to gain more speed. Alternatively, both the heel and the forefoot contact the ground in jogging. Good individual body mechanics is essential to be an injury-free sprinter.

Types of injuries sustained by sprinters usually affect the lower limbs or the lumbar spine. Muscle strains, achilles and hamstring problems and sciatica are the most commonly occurring injuries.

Most reasons for injury are the same as for joggers, particularly training when fatigued, but some do differ. Sprinters of short or middle distance tend to train in one direction only when they are in track season. Ideally training sessions should incorporate interval work both in a straight line and anti-clockwise as well as clockwise while in track season.

Commonly asked questions

Sometimes, when sprinters leave the block, for instance in a 100 metre event, it is not uncommon for them to buckle over in pain. We are usually told they have ruptured a muscle — is this possible?

Unfortunately, yes, it is possible to rupture a muscle. This can indeed be excruciatingly painful. The mechanism of injury may be related to muscle tightness. Usually it is one of the hamstring muscles (at the back of the thigh) which is torn. Imbalance of strength (usually the quadriceps are too strong in relation to the hamstrings) or insufficient warm-up, are thought to be the other most common causes.

Another reason put forward is that the neural messages from the brain do not get through quickly enough to meet the speed of contraction required in a muscle, particularly when coming out of the blocks. Conclusive evidence to support this hypothesis is still currently being studied.

Is there any benefit in a regular jogger including sprinting in their fitness programme?

This is very dependent on the expectations of the individual. Research clearly supports that sprint work incorporated into the distance runner's programme can improve speed over long distances. The same can apply to joggers if their goal and aim is to increase their speed. Slow long distance training uses the slow twitch fibres in the body while sprinting trains the fast twitch fibres. We appear to be born with a specified number of each and while we can change fast twitch to slow twitch fibres, we can only train the number of fast twitch we already have. Therefore, to include some sprint work to maximise the effectiveness with which the fast twitch fibres can be recruited would certainly help joggers if they compete in fun runs or want to increase their general pace or reduce their times.

Checklist

- If doing interval work on the track, do sprints in a straight line as well as clockwise and anti-clockwise.
- Gradually increase the pace at which you do sprint starts. Similarly, if you are practising starting out of the blocks be careful not to overtrain. Specific weight training aimed at increasing the explosive power and strength in your muscles will markedly increase your speed. However, for joggers, heavy weights should not be lifted as the additional muscle bulk can slow one's pace.
- Have you assessed your technique and style? Muscle imbalance can affect the fluency of your sprinting. Video analysis can assist this.
- Are you always getting persistent and recurrent lower limb injuries? You may need orthotics — consult a podiatrist.

Warm-up: The key to minimising the chance of injury is to slowly build up and do not go straight into sprinting when cold. Jogging on the spot, forwards, backwards, sideways and knees brought high to the chest, is essential. Progress by taking longer strides. A light jog and stretching should precede all training. If sprint starts are to be practised, the speed at which they are executed should be increased slowly.

Sprinting exercise routine

  84. Quadriceps stretch
   6. Wall exercise
  91. Hamstring stretch
  80. Adductor stretch: standing/squatting
 103. Calf stretch
 106. Achilles and soleus stretch
  60. Advanced hip stretch
  61. Hip abductor stretch
  62. Advanced hip abductor stretch
  32. Latissimus dorsi/quadratus lumborum stretch
  93. Hamstring stretch: sitting
  99. Upper hamstring stretch: lying
  29. Upper back stretch
  17. Thoracic spine and shoulder mobility exercise
  21. Tricep stretch
  22. Latissimus dorsi stretch
  78. Adductor stretch and oblique strengthening
  49. Knee hug stretch
  46. Lower back release

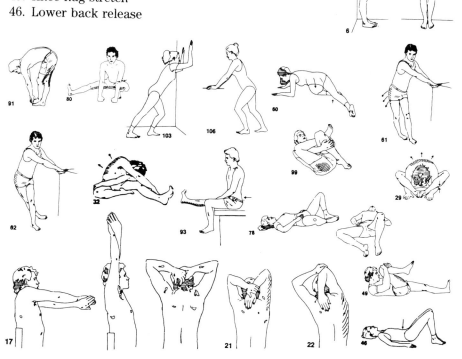

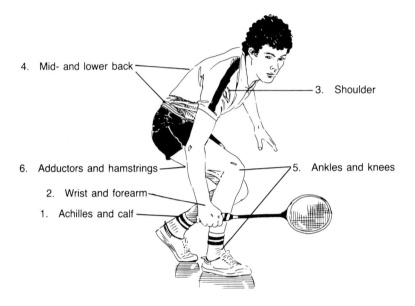

4. Mid- and lower back

3. Shoulder

6. Adductors and hamstrings

5. Ankles and knees

2. Wrist and forearm

1. Achilles and calf

SQUASH

Squash is a predominantly anaerobic activity, though for the élite, who do not take such regular breaks, it is far more aerobic.

Because of the speedy rotational movements and the jarring nature of the sport on a hard surface, lower back and calves are the most vulnerable to injury.

Most squash injuries are trauma injuries either to the eye or the ankle or simply bruises to the body from ball impact. Unnecessary muscle strains or tears may occur if the warm-up was inadequate.

Medical advice should be sought immediately any eye trauma occurs. Squash glasses to protect the eyes are highly recommended.

Treatment with ice for bruises will prevent them hardening and promote healing. A sprained ankle that has not recovered within 24 hours of ice and stretching should receive treatment. Before returning to squash, specific agility skills (change of direction and shuttle sprints), balance and peroneals strengthening (exercise 113) in addition to calf stretching (exercises 114 and 115) should be done. Taping the ankle prior to sport is to be recommended for 4 to 6 weeks post-injury.

Commonly asked questions

Do you think one can be too old to play squash?

Squash does tend to be a sport that is taken up or pursued by an over-40s group. This does have its risks. One problem is that many people in this group tend to only play once a week and this is their sole form of fitness activity. This places them at very high risk of not only injury but even heart attacks, which have been known to occur on the squash court.

On a less morbid level, the sad fact that our tissues are less elastic when older can be a precipitating factor to major calf or achilles injuries which commonly occur in this age group. Sometimes these structures may even rupture, particularly if inadequate warm-up has been performed before play. Treatment for such a trauma, notably a rupture, can be plaster for up to 2 months and rehabilitation for another 3 to 4 months prior to return to play, so preventative measures are a must!

The first precautionary measure if you are in an older age group and engaging in squash infrequently, is to introduce other activities, such as walking or swimming, regularly into your fitness or weekly regime. If possible, play a minimum of two games per week. One competition game per week definitely puts you at risk. Adequate stretching and warm-up, particularly in cold weather, while time-consuming, can lessen the risk of being out of the game altogether for 6 months or so with a ruptured muscle.

Checklist

- Protective eye glasses are highly recommended.
- Size of racquet grip is also important.
- Supportive squash shoes are a must. Make sure they do not mark the playing surface.
- Adequately hydrate your body prior to playing and replace fluid during and after play.
- If you are over 35 get a medical check-up, and pay particular attention to warming-up and stretching before you play. A fitness or stress test can give you even more detail about your current fitness level and what your physical expectations should be.

Warm-up: Should include large swinging and circular movements of the arms, practice serves, and slower pace hitting. Put your hands on your knees and rotate them to the right, then the left, two to three times. Stretching should include the shoulder, forearm and back muscles, the hamstrings, calves, ankles and knees.

Squash exercise routine

22. Latissimus dorsi stretch
21. Tricep stretch
17. Thoracic spine and shoulder mobility exercise
18. Thoracic spine and shoulder mobility exercise using a rod
31. Upper back and posterior shoulder stretch: standing
32. Latissimus dorsi/quadratus lumborum stretch
33. Side trunk stretch
19. Shoulder and scapula mobility

81. Adductor stretch: sitting
99. Upper hamstring stretch: lying
86. Hip flexor stretch
91. Hamstring stretch: standing
49. Knee hug stretch
61. Hip abductor stretch
62. Advanced hip abductor stretch
103. Calf stretch
106. Achilles and soleus stretch

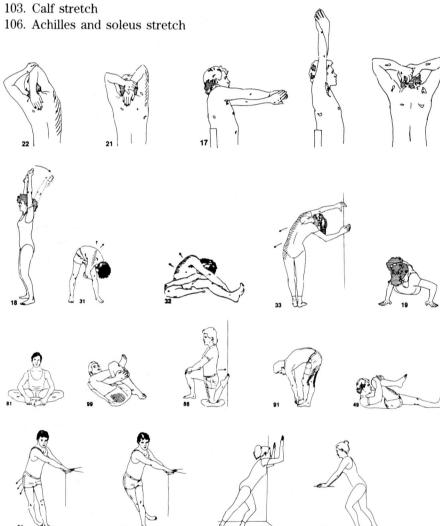

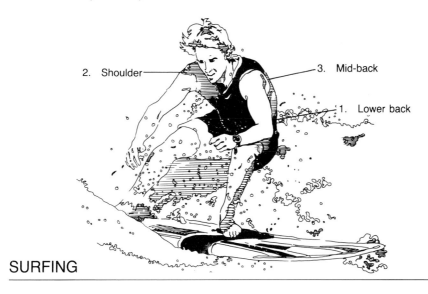

2. Shoulder

3. Mid-back

1. Lower back

SURFING

Both body surfing and board riding are excellent sports. The latter requires flexibility, agility, balance, co-ordination and, dependent on the surf, can be beneficial for cardiovascular fitness. Sitting on a board in a flat surf will not assist fitness but a taxing surf certainly makes the body work.

Board riders tend to be rather injury free, though this does not always apply to the élite rider who competes. Main problem areas tend to be stiffness in the thoracic sprine, sore shoulders and lower back pain. The first two problems can be minimised by regular stretching while the latter is usually due to lower back stiffness because of the body needing to lie in an arched position on the board, often for extended periods of time.

Checklist

- Even though surfing for most is a fun sport, being more flexible and agile and being more aerobically fit can reduce your risk of recurrent minor muscle injuries. If you have shoulder pain after surfing it may mean you are tight in your pectoral muscles and have slightly rounded shoulders. Be sure to assess your posture, so that you can identify the appropriate exercises to correct this. Jogging regularly is an ideal way to establish a basic level of fitness for surfing.

Warm-up: A light jog along the beach, and general arm loosening exercises followed by stretching regularly could prevent unnecessary injuries or muscle soreness. Main areas requiring stretching are the shoulders, mid-, upper and lower back, the hip flexors, the quadriceps and the hamstrings.

Surfing exercise routine

22. Latissimus dorsi stretch
21. Tricep stretch
17. Thoracic spine and shoulder mobility exercise
18. Thoracic spine and shoulder mobility exercise using a rod
91. Hamstring stretch: standing
49. Knee hug stretch
30. Posterior shoulder and thoracic spine stretch: sitting
29. Upper back stretch
31. Upper back and posterior shoulder stretch: standing
34. Advanced thoracic spine mobility
32. Latissimus dorsi/quadratus lumborum stretch
52. Spinal rotation stretch: sitting
81. Adductor stretch: sitting
93. Hamstring stretch: sitting
85. Quadriceps stretch and hip mobility: lying

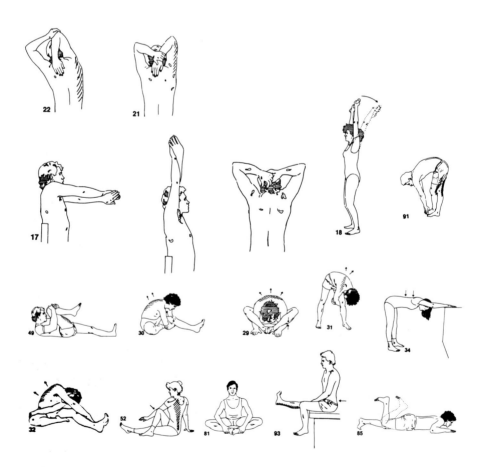

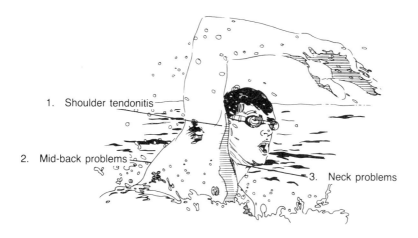

1. Shoulder tendonitis
2. Mid-back problems
3. Neck problems

SWIMMING

Swimming is an ideal activity for anyone. Because the body is supported in the water any weight-bearing stresses are totally negated. Therefore, any skeletal problems are not significant when one is in the water, though muscle balance is still important and, if ideal, will improve your efficiency. Swimming is an ideal sport for all-round fitness. It uses all the large muscle groups, therefore it helps tone muscles, builds up stamina and improves heart and lung function. It can also retain flexibility. The main injuries swimmers suffer usually affect the shoulders, the mid- or the lower back.

People who swim a lot tend to bulk up on all the anterior muscles of the chest wall. This causes tightness of these muscles especially pectoralis major and minor and leads to stress on the underlying glenohumeral (shoulder) joint. The commonest problem is tendonitis (often called 'swimmer's shoulder'). Because of the internally rotated position the humerii are in, this causes impingement or inflammation of the tendons that ride anteriorly through the joint. The biceps and supraspinatus are the most commonly affected tendons.

Preventative measures for the shoulders are to balance the type of strokes being done, particularly important for people doing a lot of freestyle or butterfly. Reviewing the number of laps one is doing is also important. Excessive lap training in preparation for a sprint (50 or 100 metre) event is not appropriate. While a sound level of aerobic fitness is certainly essential, specific training incorporating interval work (involving sprints, rest or slower laps, sprints) for sprinting events would markedly reduce the injury rate for swimmers.

A final point is that many problems swimmers have are due to poor technique. If freestyle is your major stroke try to learn to breathe bilaterally as opposed to just moving the head in the one direction. Lessons from a coach, no matter what your age, can assist technique and make swimming more enjoyable if you are not a good swimmer.

Commonly asked questions

Is any one stroke better than another?

For maximum effectiveness and to ensure muscle balance, swimming a variety of strokes is preferable to using just one. Breaststroke is especially good for the upper arms, chest, inner thighs, hips and knees; freestyle builds up the arms, shoulders, stomach and legs; backstroke is excellent for shoulder flexibility and toning of the upper arms and legs; butterfly strengthens the entire upper torso and shoulders as well as the hips, thighs and stomach. If you swim predominantly freestyle, try to loosen the shoulders in the opposite direction by finishing off with backstroke. This stroke is particularly good for strengthening the upper back muscles, the most important muscles required to maintain ideal postural alignment of the neck and shoulders. If you are specialising in one stroke for competition, weight-training is recommended to maintain balance in all muscle groups.

Is swimming good for back problems? It is so often advocated as a remedy.

Because our lifestyle for the most part is so sedentary, the load on our lower back is continuous with either sitting or standing. Therefore, swimming can be ideal for releasing this stress that our body gets subjected to daily.

Water buoyancy often permits people with back pain to exercise with minimal discomfort. This in turn will improve blood supply and promote healing, in addition to maintaining fitness.

Other weight-bearing activities such as jogging may aggravate the back complaint. Always work within pain limits though and avoid strokes which make the pain feel worse, either while swimming or afterwards. Just simply doing exercises in the water (as is done in aquarobics) will also help loosen the body, keep it supple and maintain a basic level of fitness. Consult with a specialist though if back pain persists throughout swimming.

Checklist

- Be sure to invest in a cap, goggles and ear plugs. Your swim will be much more enjoyable.
- If you are not enjoying swimming or are getting stiff muscles after you swim, check with an instructor to see if you can improve your technique. Consider introducing aquarobics into your weekly programme. Vary the stroke you use when you have a swim. Introduce some faster and slower laps to be more effective in your workout. Try not to stop too long at the end of the pool after each lap, or you will reduce the effectiveness of your cardiovascular workout.
- Stretch before and after each swim to prevent muscle soreness, particularly the shoulders and upper and mid-back. Be sure to assess your posture and incorporate the appropriate exercises in your daily routine if you think you are developing round shoulders.

Warm-up: Loosen the shoulders and arms with large circular swinging movements both forward and back. Pull each knee up to the chest and then behind to loosen the hamstrings and quadriceps. Use the walls near the pool to do side trunk stretches. Stretches for the shoulders, upper back and legs should follow. Do a lap slowly to get the circulation going through the body and repeat these stretches using the pool wall at each end to assist you. This is particularly helpful for the lower back and shoulders. If you swim competitively, do not just warm-up 2 hours prior to your event. Try to loosen up and stretch as close to your event as possible.

Swimming exercise routine

1. Neck flexion
2. Neck extension
3. Neck rotation
4. Neck side flexion
22. Latissimus dorsi stretch
21. Tricep stretch
28. Thoracic spine and rhomboids stretch
17. Thoracic spine and shoulder mobility exercise
18. Thoracic spine and shoulder mobility exercise using a rod
31. Upper back and posterior shoulder stretch: standing
34. Advanced thoracic spine mobility
24. Shoulder rotation: lying
50. Spinal rotation stretch: lying
93. Hamstring stretch: sitting
32. Latissimus dorsi/quadratus lumborum stretch
33. Side trunk stretch
80. Adductor stretch: standing/squatting
86. Hip flexor stretch
49. Knee hug stretch
98. Upper hamstring stretch
61. Hip abductor stretch
62. Advanced hip abductor stretch
117. Ankle mobility

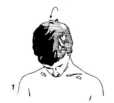

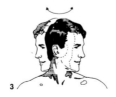
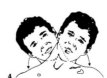

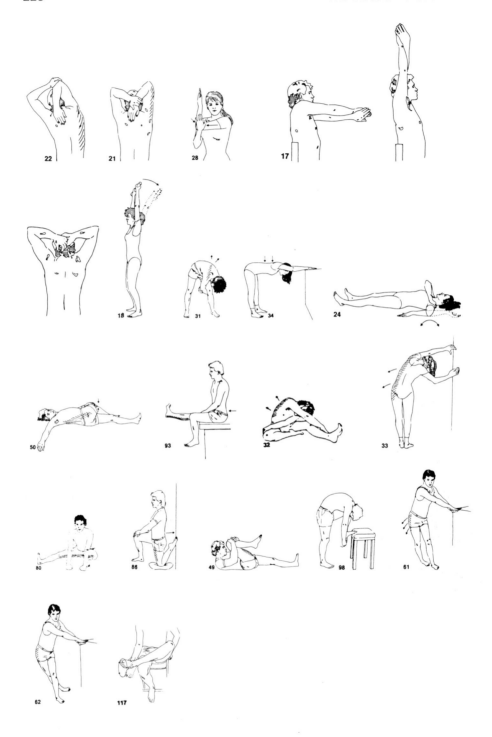

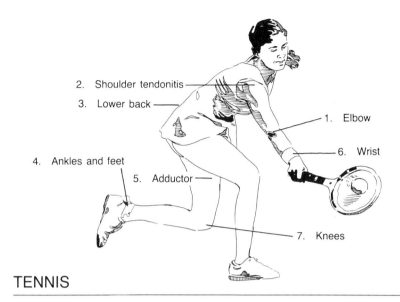

2. Shoulder tendonitis

3. Lower back

1. Elbow

6. Wrist

4. Ankles and feet

5. Adductor

7. Knees

TENNIS

The main skills required for tennis are agility, co-ordination, timing, and flexibility of all major muscle groups, upper and lower limb and the torso. Good stamina will also enhance your enjoyment of the game.

Because of the rotational, stretching and twisting movements required in this sport, shoulder, lower back, calf and ankle problems are the main injuries seen. Elbow problems are also common. Most problems are related to poor technique, inadequate flexibility or muscle imbalance.

Adequate flexibility and review of technique, particularly of your serve, if it is a lower back complaint, can reduce your chances of injury.

One of the most common problems for tennis players is termed 'tennis elbow'. This is the name for pain on the lateral aspect of the elbow. It may refer to a multitude of conditions though tendonitis and bursitis are the two most common. (See Baseball.) Sometimes any condition affecting the elbow is given the general term of tennis elbow or the medical term medial epicondylitis — both simply meaning inflammation around the elbow.

The main reasons for the problem occurring are poor technique, incorrect grip size, too heavy a racquet and muscle imbalance around the shoulder, elbow and forearm. Other contributing factors may be the frequency of play, age and sex and poor levels of conditioning and fitness.

Some preventative measures are listed below.

Technique Trying to slice or spin the ball particularly on the backhand shot or while serving stresses the forearm muscles which arise from the elbow. Blocking the backhand rather than using a full swing-back and follow-through can also stress the elbow by jarring this joint at the time of impact with the ball. Other than these most obvious points, regular review of your style and technique by a coach can not only improve your tennis standard but also prevent bad habits predisposing you to injuries.

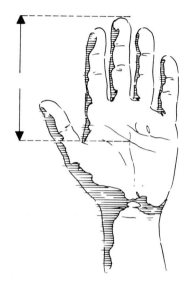

8.5   Grip size
Measure from the tip of the middle finger to the middle crease line in the palm of your
hand.

Grip size If your grip size is too small there is a tendency to grip the racquet
too hard when you play. To determine your grip size note the above diagram.

Measure from the tip of the middle finger to middle crease line in your palm.
This should equal the grip size you select.

Racquet choice A racquet too light, too heavy or strung too tightly can add to
forearm stress. Graphite absorbs shock better than other materials and mid-size
is usually recommended to reduce the stress created by miss-hits. Weight is
important also. Muscle fatigue and injury can be caused by a heavy racquet. The
average weight of the lighter racquet best suited to recreational players is
approximately 350 grams. String tension is also significant for reducing stress on
the elbow. Tension too tight allows greater impact, and shock forces to be trans-
mitted to the forearm. The tension recommended in normal racquets is between
25–27 kilograms. Oversized racquets require more initial tension to allow for
the increase in area.

Other preventative measures

- Adequate regular stretching, particularly elbow, calves, hamstrings, adductors, shoulders and lower back, so that good technique is able to be exercised
  without jarring the elbow.
- Do not overtrain or overpractise one particular skill — do not do an entire
  practice session of serving. Do some general stroke work as well.
- Warm-up slowly. Do not hit the hardest ball or do your strongest serve first.
- Aim for consistency and fluency in play before working on technique.

- Review your technique regularly.
- Review your postural mechanics.
- Do specific elbow stretches if you get elbow stiffness after tennis. Do not use an elasticated band over the elbow. If you do find an elbow guard eases a chronic problem you have, pay particular attention to stretching the muscles under the guard, as they are not able to work through their full range. When possible give yourself breaks occasionally from wearing the support — though *do not* play through pain.

Checklist

Are you always playing on hard or pexiplave surfaces? Try to vary this with grass or sand surfaces. The least stressful on the body is synthetic grass.

Have you chosen the correct size and weight racquet? Grip size, tension of strings, type of strings, and what your racquet is made of, are all important considerations. Graphite is recommended, and a mid-size racquet is also good. Are your shoes well-supported, cushioned and designed for multi-directional movement? Replace them when they get too old.

Is it time to review your skills? Tennis requires balance, precision timing, co-ordination and agility. Are you practising all these? Are you fit, flexible and strong enough? Being aerobically fitter will mean you fatigue in a match less readily.

Are you preparing your body adequately prior to play? Are you over or under-training or playing? Playing once only per week puts you at risk. Try to incorporate some other form of aerobic fitness into your weekly regime such as jogging, or aerobics. Are you too overdeveloped on your dominant side, particularly in your back? This can create imbalance and cause potential problems.

Tennis exercise routine

  6. Wall exercise
  1. Neck flexion
  2. Neck extension
  3. Neck rotation
  4. Neck side flexion
 22. Latissimus dorsi stretch
 21. Tricep stretch
 17. Thoracic spine and shoulder mobility exercise
 18. Thoracic spine and shoulder mobility exercise using a rod
 31. Upper back and posterior shoulder stretch: standing
 34. Advanced thoracic spine mobility
 41. Lower back stretch
 32. Latissimus dorsi/quadratus lumborum stretch
 33. Side trunk stretch
 94. Hamstring and lower back stretch

86. Hip flexor stretch
80. Adductor stretch: standing/squatting
103. Calf stretch
106. Achilles and soleus stretch
27. Wrist and finger stretch

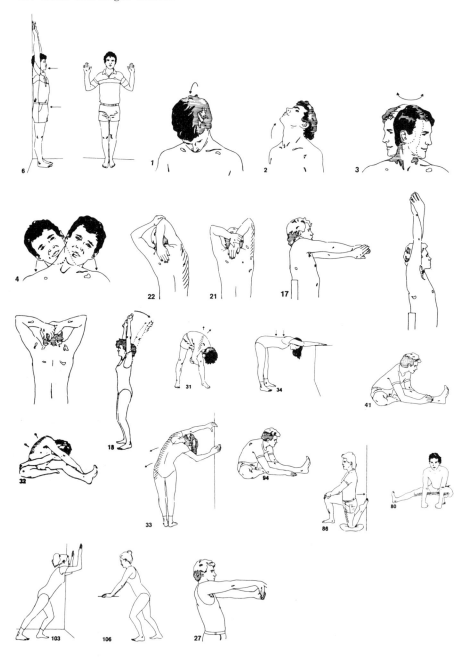

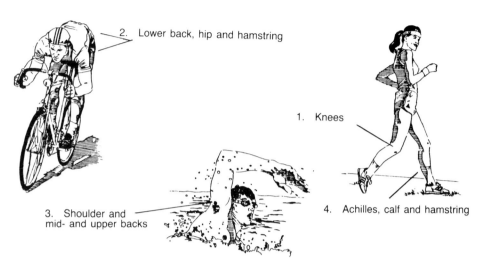

2. Lower back, hip and hamstring

1. Knees

3. Shoulder and mid- and upper backs

4. Achilles, calf and hamstring

TRIATHLONS

Certainly this physically demanding sport has become very popular these last 4 to 5 years. The combination of swimming, running and cycling can place heavy demands on the body's musculoskeletal system. So if you are continually getting injured when you first choose this sport — you may need to rethink your choice.

Problem areas are usually the elbows, wrists, mid- and upper back, lower back, knees, tight hamstrings and calves. The major reason for injury is over-training. Try to join a triathlon club where you are able to discuss the various ways to train for this event.

The physical training required to be at peak fitness for all three sports is intense. Once you have decided how to schedule your week to fit in training for each of these activities you need to continually reassess your programme to be sure it is best suited for your individual needs. That is, are the distances you are training sufficient? What is your immediate goal (or competition) or your long term goal? Are the demands on your body too much?

If you are continually tired and run-down or always getting minor injuries, it may be that you are overtraining. It is critical to do overall stretching for the body daily to minimise your predisposition to injury. Consult an experienced triathloner or sports specialist to design a programme catering for your specific needs and requirements.

Checklist

- Are you training on a variety of terrains with your running?
- Do not just practise in a pool if the swimming section of your competition is in open water. Try to acclimatise to this situation where the water may be very cold and muddy.
- Is your bicycle suited to your individual needs? (See Cycling.)

- Be sure you have a wetsuit that keeps you warm but does not permit you to get too hot. Wear practical clothes so you can change quickly between each sport.
- If you are stronger in some sports than in others, be careful not to neglect the others, as this will increase your risk of injury when you do compete.
- Set your goals realistically when you are training for competition. Be careful not to overtrain.
- Try to train with friends and get them to keep a check on your technique and style in all three sports. Obvious problems can often be overlooked when you train by yourself.
- If you are injury prone, consult a sports specialist to screen for musculo-skeletal imbalances before considering changing your choice of sport.
- For any of these sports, consult a specialist at the first sign of pain or injury. Left untreated, chronic problems will develop quickly.

Warm-up: For all three sports the extent and length of your warm-up will depend on the intensity of your workout session. For each activity loosen up the shoulders with large circular movements. For swimming use a wall to assist with your stretching. For running and cycling place extra emphasis on your stretches once you have completed your workout (include them in your cool-down). Stretching prior to your activity is also important.

Triathlon exercise routine

  22. Latissimus dorsi stretch
  21. Tricep stretch
  17. Thoracic spine and shoulder mobility exercise
  18. Thoracic spine and shoulder mobility exercise using a rod
  32. Latissimus dorsi/quadratus lumborum stretch
  33. Side trunk stretch
  24. Shoulder rotation: lying
  93. Hamstring stretch: sitting
  29. Upper back stretch
  30. Posterior shoulder and thoracic spine stretch: sitting
  41. Lower back stretch
  49. Knee hug stretch
  78. Adductor stretch and oblique strengthening
  60. Advanced hip stretch
  80. Adductor stretch: standing/squatting
  86. Hip flexor stretch
103. Calf stretch
106. Achilles and soleus stretch
  36. Cat stretch: extension
  37. Cat stretch: flexion
  38. Lower back release

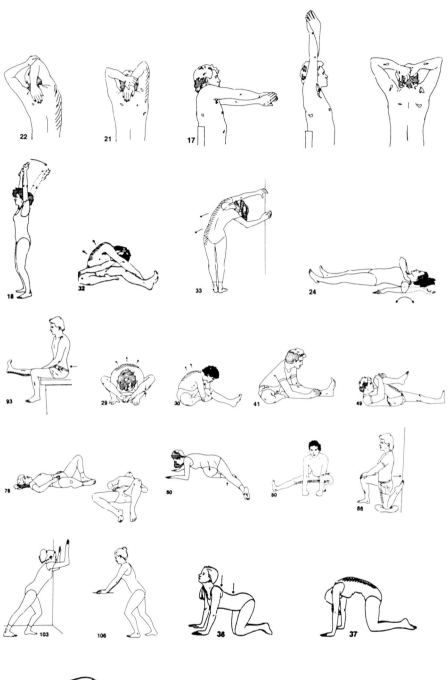

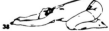

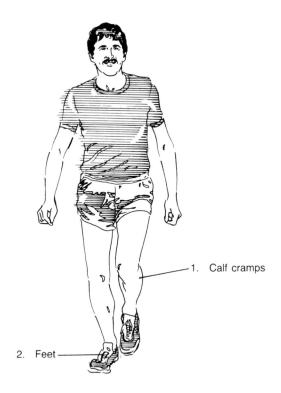

1. Calf cramps

2. Feet

WALKING

Walking is the ideal activity for any person no matter what age, height or weight.

However, a leisurely stroll will achieve little. Walking at a brisk pace (6–11 kilometres per hour) will tax the heart and lungs more effectively to gain cardiovascular fitness. It is best to set yourself a goal. For instance, increase the distance that you walk in one week while the next week try to decrease the time at which you walk this distance. Take deep breaths while you are walking to fill your lungs to their capacity and increase the effectiveness of your activity. Stretching and doing arm exercises while you walk will enhance your workout still further. Try to find a friend or a group of people to walk with. This will make your exercise so much more enjoyable and more fun. Be sure that you can carry on a conversation or that you can 'whistle while you walk'. This is a helpful guideline to ensure you are not stressing yourself too much. Do not forget the three Ss (see page 55) and the ideals of getting fit using the FITT formula. (See page 26 .)

Injuries are minimal but buying yourself a good pair of walking shoes will reduce any potential problems that could occur.

For walking, jogging shoes are probably better than a tennis or squash shoe.

(For details refer to Jogging.) However, many good walking shoes are available on the market. The key features to look for are a strong heel counter, forefoot flexibility, mid-foot support and a good arch support.

In addition to the above, the shoe when you buy it should feel supportive but *not tight*. Try to buy shoes in the afternoon when your feet may be swollen after the day's activities.

Checklist

- A supportive pair of walking shoes is essential for brisk walking. Jogging shoes are preferable to tennis or squash shoes. Comfortable, loose-fitting clothes should be worn so the body is free to move quickly. Wear a hat to prevent heat exhaustion in the summer months.
- Try to include hills in your walk, and vary the surface and direction you take when you walk.
- Keep a check of your pulse to check you are working aerobically.
- Try to walk briskly and go with a group of friends where possible.
- You should adopt a comfortable heel-toe gait when you walk and relax the shoulders as you walk briskly.

Warm-up: Ideally your warm-up should be incorporated into your walk. For the first few minutes start your walk at a leisurely pace and do a general warm-up of the upper limb by doing large swinging and circular movements of the arms. Then do the stretches at the end of this section before you proceed with your brisk walking workout. Shake the legs free when you have finished stretching.

Walking exercise routine

22. Latissimus dorsi stretch
17. Thoracic spine and shoulder mobility exercise
18. Thoracic spine and shoulder mobility exercise using a rod
33. Side trunk stretch
84. Quadriceps stretch
98. Upper hamstring stretch
80. Adductor stretch: standing/squatting
91. Hamstring stretch: standing
93. Hamstring stretch: sitting
117. Ankle mobility
61. Hip abductor stretch
62. Advanced hip abductor stretch
103. Calf stretch
106. Achilles and soleus stretch
107. Deep toe flexor stretch
50. Spinal rotation: lying

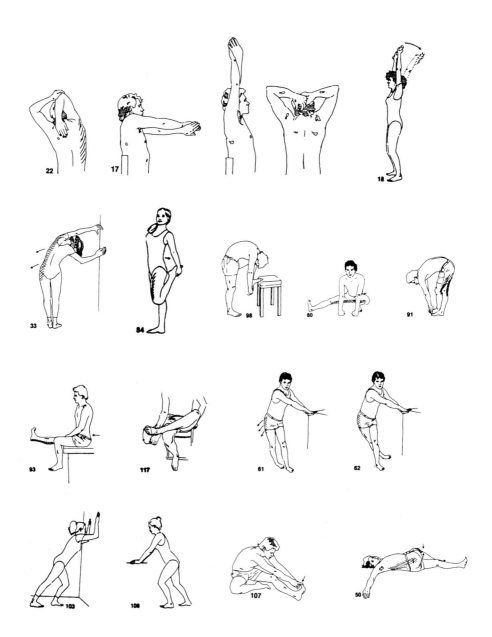

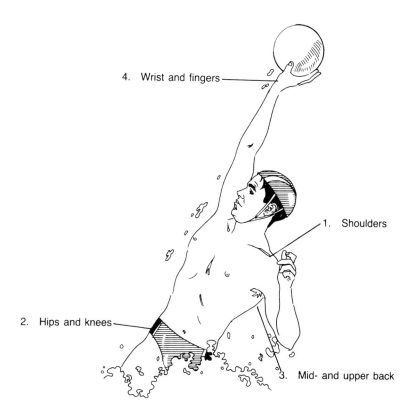

4. Wrist and fingers

1. Shoulders

2. Hips and knees

3. Mid- and upper back

WATERPOLO

The strength and agility required for this sport is often underrated. Strength in the shoulder, upper back, forearms, fingers and wrists is imperative to develop adequate ball handling skills.

The sport itself is predominantly an anaerobic activity because players are replaced regularly throughout a match. However, an improved level of aerobic fitness will certainly reduce the onset of fatigue often brought on by exercising in the water.

Waterpolo tends to be a highly competitive contact sport. Theoretically it is meant to be a predominantly non-contact sport but players soon learn this is not usually the case.

Main problem areas tend to be the shoulders, neck, mid- and upper back, hips, knees and lower back. Reasons for injury are usually related to muscle tightness or muscle imbalance particularly of the anterior chest muscles (the pectorals) and the hip flexors (iliopsoas).

Therefore loosening up all major muscle groups and warming-up well before both training and match play as well as stretching regularly in between playing sessions is critical.

Stretching of the shoulders should include all muscles which contribute to shoulder functioning, in particular the pectorals, anterior deltoid, latissimus dorsi and trapezii. Shoulder tendonitis may develop if muscle imbalance develops around the shoulder joint.

The other area of focus should be around the hip joint. Because of the continual rotatory action of the legs while in the water, hip problems, often presenting as groin pain, are quite common. Improved flexibility of the hip musculature, particularly iliopsoas, adductors and the quadriceps, can reduce the risk of these lower limb problems developing.

Strength in the legs is also very important to all players to assist with the explosive power required when jumping out of the water to catch the ball, particularly so for the goal keeper. Weight training aimed at developing strength in the hip flexors, abductors and the hip extensors can assist minimising fatigue and maximising powerful play.

Checklist

- You need to assess posture regularly to ensure round shoulders do not develop from overdevelopment and shortening of the pectoral muscles in the chest. Pay particular attention to the hip flexors and adductors to prevent hip pain from developing.
- Try to maintain a basic level of aerobic fitness by doing some other form of aerobic activity. Obviously swimming is the most appropriate and convenient choice. Try to incorporate some speed work by doing fast and slow laps in your training sessions.
- Swimming a few lengths of the pool incorporating as many styles as one can do (such as freestyle, or backstroke), will loosen the body a little prior to your stretching. Using the edge of the pool for stretching against can increase the effectiveness of your stretching. Ball handling skills should also be practised prior to match play so that the body can adjust to the jarring that occurs in the shoulder joint itself during play.

Waterpolo exercise routine

1. Neck flexion
2. Neck extension
3. Neck rotation
4. Neck side flexion
22. Latissimus dorsi stretch
21. Tricep stretch
18. Thoracic spine and shoulder mobility using towel instead of rod
26. Wrist, shoulder and neck stretch
30. Posterior shoulder and thoracic spine stretch: sitting *OR*
31. Upper back and posterior shoulder stretch: standing
34. Advanced thoracic spine mobility
33. Side trunk stretch
84. Quadriceps stretch

61. Hip abductor stretch
62. Advanced hip abductor stretch
98. Upper hamstring stretch
49. Knee hug stretch
19. Shoulder and scapula mobility
93. Hamstring stretch: sitting
91. Hamstring stretch: standing
97. Combined hamstring and adductor stretch
 6. Wall exercise (Use this exercise to check and see if the shoulders are tightening up too much.)

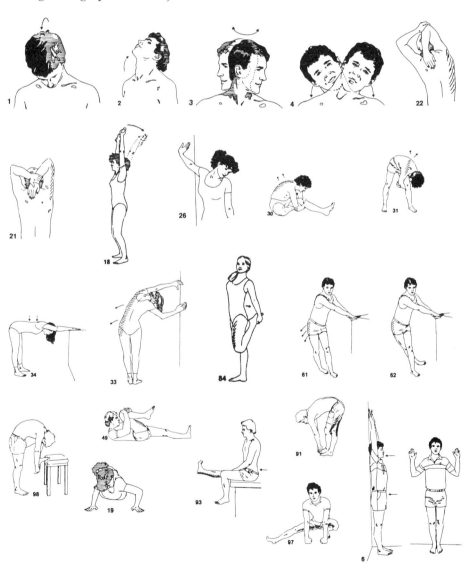

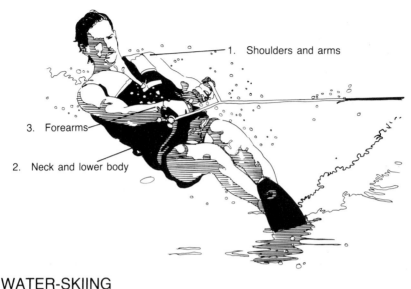

1. Shoulders and arms

3. Forearms

2. Neck and lower body

WATER-SKIING

While predominantly a recreational activity for most of us, the fun of water-skiing can be spoilt if injuries or muscle stiffness recur too often.

The main problem areas are the arms, shoulders, mid- and upper back, the thighs and hips, apart from unexpected traumas associated with falls.

Checklist

- If you are a beginner, do not try anything too potentially harmful. Work up slowly to using one ski. Being daring can lead to major injury. Wear a life jacket at all times. Wear a wetsuit at all times. This will not only keep you warm but also protect you a little when you fall.

Warm-up: While not the ideal situation and location is often not conducive to doing an adequate warm-up, it is far from ideal to jump straight onto a pair of skis and go skiing. The more tense the body is the harder it will hit the water — if you do fall! It doesn't matter how warm or cold it is, it always helps to warm-up a little.

Jumping in the water and doing some swimming and range of movement stretches in the water is usually sufficient warm-up. Alternatively a light jog prior to stretching may be possible.

Water-skiing exercise routine

22. Latissimus dorsi stretch
21. Tricep stretch
17. Thoracic spine and shoulder mobility exercise
23. Shoulder rotations: sitting

27. Wrist and finger stretch
29. Upper back stretch
49. Knee hug stretch
52. Spinal rotation stretch: sitting
60. Advanced hip stretch
93. Hamstring stretch: sitting
33. Side trunk stretch
84. Quadriceps stretch
103. Calf stretch
106. Achilles and soleus stretch

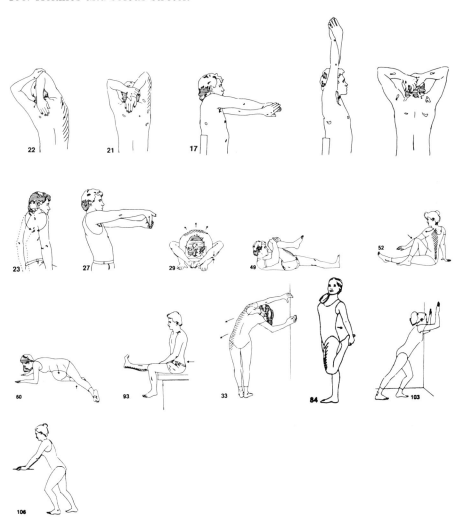

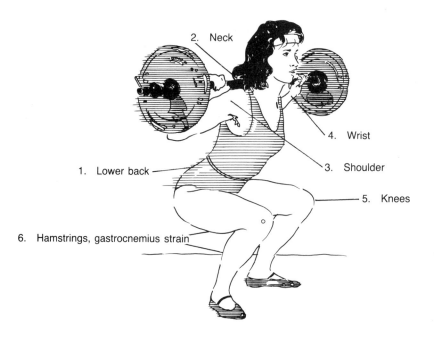

2. Neck

4. Wrist

3. Shoulder

1. Lower back

5. Knees

6. Hamstrings, gastrocnemius strain

WEIGHT TRAINING

Some people use weight training as a sport on its own while others use it as an adjunct to assist their sporting performance in their chosen sport. Working with weights often encourages repetitive contractions of a muscle often within a shortened range. Therefore, it is essential both before and after a workout to stretch, so as not to cause chronic shortening of that muscle.

Main problem areas are shoulders, knees, neck, mid- and lower back, wrists, groin and hip. The main reasons for injury are overtraining, poor form or technique while using weights, or problems related to muscle imbalance.

Aerobic fitness, strength, bulking, power or a combination of some of these can be gained from using weights. Depending on what you are aiming to achieve the following basic guidelines indicate the type of weight training necessary for the differing needs. Note these are only guidelines. You must consult a specialist to design a programme to suit your specific needs.

1. **Aerobic fitness** Weight training for aerobic fitness needs to be light and repetitions kept high (ten to fifteen is recommended, but anything up to twenty to thirty is all right). Minimal rest breaks between exercise stations to keep heart rate up is the key to working aerobically. Many gymnasiums offer circuit training classes incorporating weights. This is an excellent way of improving stamina as well as strength. This type of class involves interspersing the use of weights at one particular station with other forms of aerobic activity such as jogging on the spot, cycling or using a rebounder. The class usually lasts 25–30 minutes and is an excellent means of improving aerobic fitness while increasing muscle strength.

2. **Strength** An individually designed programme to suit your needs is a must before you take up weights to gain strength. You need to consider whether it is strength for a specific sport you need, or a specific skill (for example, to improve one's serve in tennis), or do you simply want to build up or develop an increase in overall body strength?

For strengthening there are different formulas used. The most basic of these is the use of eight to twelve repetitions starting with the first set and building up to three sets. When this is achieved comfortably and becomes too easy the weight should be increased, first for one set, then the others.

For specifically increasing muscle bulk, a basic level of strength needs to be built up before progressing to heavier weights. It is the use of very heavy weights with minimal repetitions (for instance two or three repetitions) that achieves the most effective bulking. The inverse pyramid training effect is a common method of combining strength training with the desired effects of bulking. Body builders often use this form of weight training, either part or all of it. The method uses twelve repetitions in the first set, six to eight in the second and two to three repetitions in the third set. This sequence is then repeated in reverse, increasing the weight.

3. **Power** If explosive power is desired (for example, for training for shot-put, javelin and so on), after the base level of strength has been achieved, the actual weight lifted should be kept high and repetitions should be kept low. Usually free weights incorporating the squat, bench, and clean and jerk techniques of the type used in power lifting competitions are suitable training for these sports.

Commonly asked questions

At what age is it safe to start weight training?

It is difficult to dictate a specific age as the commencement of weight training should be based on the musculoskeletal maturity of the child. While a child is in a growth spurt heavy weights should be avoided as the growth plates in the bone are very vulnerable to damage. Ligaments are very elastic in the teenager so overstretching or overloading can cause stress on underlying joints. Before the age of 13, the use of weight training is highly questionable.

Lighter weights to assist with performance and balancing out strength required in other sports (for example, rowing) may be safe in adolescent years. However, the teenager using weights must be carefully monitored. Any development of pain in a joint may indicate overload is occurring. Consult a sports specialist if you are uncertain if a child should be using weights.

If I have been weight training for some time and I stop what will happen to my muscles and skin and will I put on weight?

The dreaded thought of having flabby muscles when weight training has ceased is one that has crossed many a body builder's or weight trainer's mind!

Fortunately, the changes are not as dramatic as this. All that is lost is strength and this is lost very quickly. Within a week changes will be seen. Some body builders and people using heavy weights actually get stretch marks showing in their skin after they have neglected weights for some time — even in their biceps! Dependent upon how many years the individual has been weight training, usually there is simply a gradual reduction in the size of all muscles, and providing a general level of fitness is maintained, the dreaded 'flabby' muscle syndrome should not occur.

With respect to weight, usually weight is lost when weight-training ceases, because muscle weighs more than fat. It is a fallacy that muscle 'turns to fat' when you stop weight-training.

Checklist

- Replace free weights after doing each exercise to ensure either yourself or another doesn't trip on the weights which are lying around.
- Check equipment regularly for faulty functioning.
- Be sure to get an experienced person to design your weight-training programme so that you are using weights appropriately to meet your needs.
- Learn how to use each station and perform each exercise correctly to reduce your risk of injury. Be sure to balance your strengthening programme between all muscle groups so that unnecessary overload on joints does not occur. Establish and set your goals realistically. Remember, for some body types, for instance the ectomorph, hypertrophy of muscle cannot be so readily achieved as for other types such as the mesomorph. (See Chapter 2.) So be aware of the limitations of your body type.
- If you are using heavy free weights, it is important to always have a 'spotter'. This is another person nearby in case you cannot complete the repetitions you were attempting to do in this form of maximal training. You should use a supportive back guard to support the spine.

Warm-up: Either a light jog, using the stationary bicycle, or rowing machine, or jumping on the mini trampoline for 12–15 minutes will generally loosen up the body prior to your weights workout. It is imperative to stretch, both before and after your workout.

Weight-training exercise routine

22. Latissimus dorsi stretch
21. Tricep stretch
17. Thoracic spine and shoulder mobility exercise
18. Thoracic spine and shoulder mobility exercise using a rod
26. Wrist, shoulder and neck stretch
30. Posterior shoulders and thoracic spine stretch: sitting
11. Pectoral stretch

34. Advanced thoracic spine mobility
29. Upper back stretch
91. Hamstring stretch: standing
41. Lower back stretch
42. Advanced lower back stretch
43. Advanced lower back stretch with hip rotation
103. Calf stretch
106. Achilles and soleus stretch
80. Adductor stretch: standing/squatting
60. Advanced hip stretch
86. Hip flexor stretch
32. Latissimus dorsi/quadratus lumborum stretch
33. Side trunk stretch
94. Hamstring and lower back stretch
29. Upper back stretch
50. Spinal rotation stretch: lying
51. Double leg spinal rotation
52. Spinal rotation stretch: sitting
36. Cat stretch: extension
37. Cat stretch: flexion
38. Lower back release
49. Knee hug stretch

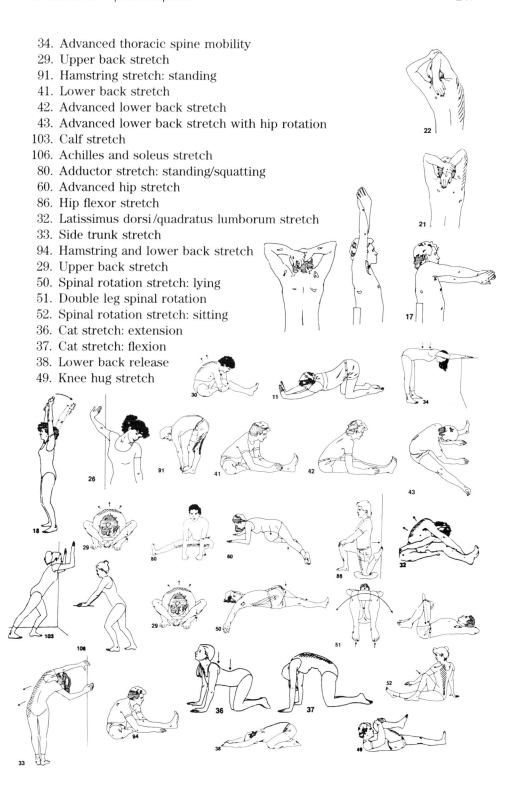

PART 3 — MUSCLE CARE

9 — WHAT TO DO IF YOU HURT A MUSCLE

Deciding whether to rest, to exercise, to consult a specialist or listen to a friend's advice when you have sore muscles or a pain, can be a dilemma. This chapter outlines self-help measures for when you injure your muscles. We will discuss the pros and cons of various methods of treatment. Firstly, though, we need to clarify some of the common terms used in relation to muscle care.

MUSCLE INJURY TERMINOLOGY

Trauma This word is used interchangeably with injury. A direct trauma is when there has been direct impact to an area. An indirect trauma is when a soft tissue (either muscle, tendon or ligament) is injured or damaged without impact to the area, for instance, a muscle strain.

Acute This refers to an injury which occurred recently, usually during the last 2–3 days.

Chronic This refers to an injury that has been present in the body for more than a few weeks.

Haematoma A bruise.

Contusion Where a bruise has started to consolidate in an area. For instance, this can happen with a corked thigh.

Muscle strain Refers to a tear of some of the myofibrils of the muscle. Repetitive stress over a period of time on a specific area may cause microtrauma to any part of the musculotendinous unit (for instance, a chronic hamstring strain), while a macrotrauma refers to one specific injury to an area (such as a corked thigh). Muscle strains are usually classified as first, second or third degree depending on the severity of the injury. Muscle strains which recover in 2–10 days are usually said to be a first degree strain. A third degree strain is used to describe a ruptured muscle.

Muscle soreness Refers to the stiffness which occurs after doing unfamiliar or excessive exercise. It usually does not occur until 24 hours after the activity and peaks at 48 hours. It should be gone by 72 hours. If it does not then it is probably a muscle strain or some other related injury.

251

Ligament sprain This is when a ligament is overstretched. It is again classified as a first to third degree strain. A first degree is a partial tear of some of the fibres of the ligament (for example, a sprained ankle) and takes 4–6 weeks to totally repair itself, though with taping for support, return to sport is usually possible earlier than this. A third degree sprain refers to a ruptured ligament. This is common in the knee and requires surgical repair within 7–10 days following the injury in most instances. Conservative treatment, meaning strengthening exercises and physiotherapeutic modalities, may sometimes be used, depending on which ligament is ruptured, how actively engaged in sport the person is, and so on.

Musculoligamentous injury This occurs when both the muscle and the ligament are damaged in an area. It is common in the neck or back after a car accident or when injury occurs from heavy lifting.

Tendonitis 'Itis' refers to inflammation, so tendonitis refers to inflammation of a tendon. Most tendons are enclosed within a sheath and the tendon becomes inflamed within the sheath with repetitive stress or abnormal loading. Shoulder tendonitis is common if imbalance of muscles exists around the shoulder causing impingement of tendons such as the biceps or supraspinatus muscle. The achilles tendon does not have a sheath right around it but it has a covering, on one side only. If it becomes inflamed, this is known as peritendonitis.

Bursitis Inflammation of the bursa. This is a fluid-filled sac made of connective tissue which lies between bone and tendon to prevent friction occurring with movement. It becomes inflamed with abnormal loading (due to muscle imbalance) or through overexercising a specific area.

Capsulitis This refers to inflammation of the surface of a synovial joint. It is common in the hip or shoulder.

THE RICE(D) PRINCIPLE

The immediate action to take when acute trauma occurs is to use ice in accordance with the RICE(D) principle. Basically this means:

R = Rest Be sure to take the load or weight off the injured area. If trauma has been painful do not keep exercising.

I = Ice Apply ice as soon as possible. This can be done by wrapping fresh ice in a damp towel, using a commercially made ice pack, a bag of frozen peas, or filling a paper cup with water and freezing it, then massaging it on the affected area.

C = Compression Apply a compression (stretch) bandage to the area to prevent excessive swelling. Do not use non-elastic tape.

E = **Elevation** Try to keep the injured area elevated to permit gravity to assist reduction of swelling.

D = **Diagnosis** Consult a doctor, physiotherapist or other specialist if pain and swelling do not settle within 24 hours, to receive a professional diagnosis and advice regarding your complaint.

ICE VERSUS HEAT TREATMENT

When we traumatise soft tissue, bleeding occurs in the area. If the muscle fibres are damaged, the normal physiological muscle pump which assists the movement of blood from peripheral areas to more central regions is impeded, and swelling from a traumatised area is not effectively removed. Ice has a local effect of closing down blood vessels (vasoconstriction) which prevents excessive bleeding. A response in the hypothalamus of the brain (called a hypothalamic response) responds to this local vasoconstriction and sends blood to the deeper vessels to counteract this effect. Mild vasodilation (opening up of blood vessels) occurs, and this extra flow deep to the area assists to reduce swelling as more fluid is pumped back to the heart. Vasoconstriction then reoccurs which causes a mild pumping effect in the soft tissue. All this takes place in 10–14 minutes.

Ice should be applied for a minimum of 10–15 minutes. For larger areas apply it for a little longer.

For an acutely sprained ankle an ice bucket may be used. This consists of ice cubes in water. Immerse the swollen limb and when it is numb take it out and start flexing and extending the foot. Keep repeating this for 10–15 minutes every 2 hours till the severe swelling has subsided.

In an acute injury, while there is any sign of bleeding, heat should not be used as it causes vasodilation which increases the bleeding. For most sprains it is fine to use heat after 72 hours. However, acute traumas such as partially torn hamstrings, where bruising is present in the entire muscle belly, until yellowing of the bruise begins to show, indicating healing, *do not use heat!* In this instance, as well as others (such as a corked thigh), ice may need to be used for up to a week — even longer.

OINTMENTS AND RUBS

Scientific research to support the effectiveness of many of the lubricants currently available on the market is lacking. However, if we analyse most of these products and how they work, their role seems less questionable. Most heat rubs contain the substance methyl salicylate, a derivative of ethyl salicylate which forms the basis of aspirin (used to reduce inflammation). Methyl salycilate is also the commercial name for wintergreen oil, a centuries-old remedy for use on muscle aches and pains.

Heat rubs cause a counter-irritant effect on the skin. This creates a superficial chemical reaction giving rise to redness and warmth in the skin locally and a subsequent increased blood flow to the area. This local response is claimed to assist with circulation deeper to the area. To what extent this is achieved is as yet inconclusive.

What we do know is that heat rubs do provide a mild analgesic effect. Most people use heat rubs because of this and also because of the warmth in the area produced once it has been applied. Both before sport and after sport, heat rubs may be used. The rubs should not be used to replace warm-up and stretches, but used on a painful area and combined with massage can provide considerable relief to mild muscular aches or pains, particularly post-exercise muscle soreness.

Never use heat rubs on the face, under the arm or in the groin area. It is safe to apply these rubs several times each day.

COMMONLY ASKED QUESTIONS

Should I exercise if I have a cold or viral infection?

When your body is carrying some form of infection the best way to assist it to fight this and promote the healing process is to sleep whenever possible or just simply rest. If you have a temperature this is even more important. Also, colds tend to afflict us more when we are run down physically — maybe you were overtraining? Therefore, respect the body and re-evaluate your fitness (or lifestyle) programme. Viral infections often affect the nervous system so if you exercise you may feel worse afterwards. Let your body have a few days' rest if you are feeling tired or run down, or if you have an infection in your body. When you do return to your sport or activity it will be much more enjoyable and not so stressful.

Will supports which keep an area warm help my injury?

There are many supports available that are not guards to protect an area, but when worn keep an area warm. The physiological mechanism of how these guards work is difficult to explain. It seems some type of counter-irritant effect is again provided improving blood supply to the area. For chronic muscle stiffness and strains past their acute phase, many athletes find these supports very helpful for keeping an area warm. Providing accurate diagnosis has been made eliminating a major problem, and the causes for why an injury has occurred have been ascertained, the use of these types of supports to maintain warmth in an area is recommended. Corked thighs and tight hamstrings are examples of injuries where these supports may be of benefit to the player.

When I have sore muscles after exercise should I rest or continue with exercise?

If you have stiff, sore muscles from doing unfamiliar or excessive exercise, it is best to stretch and do some lighter exercise. Rest will only tighten your muscles further. However, controversy does surround the answer to this question.

Why do I get stitches and cramps when I run?

Scientific reasons are lacking for stitches in the abdomen, and even the anterior shoulder, or cramps in the abdomen or lower limb.

It was previously thought that cramps were due to a lack of salt in the body. This has since been found not to be the case. Our western diet provides adequate levels of sodium (salt) to dispel this hypothesis.

The current explanation for cramps is dehydration, that is, inadequate fluid in the body prior to exercising. Before any vigorous exercise session, an increase in fluid intake (two to three glasses of water) is recommended. Do not drink strong salt-based drinks as this will have a counter-productive effect. Weak drinks of this nature are not a problem.

Another theory for abdominal cramps is that they are caused by milk-based products, which are very slow to digest, and may be taken too soon before an exercise session. You will need to minimise the intake of these types of food prior to exercise to know if this is what is causing the cramping.

In the case of stitches, clinical findings outweigh any scientific theory. In the author's clinical experience, a small section of fibritic tissue or muscle spasm in the diaphragm or of the iliopsoas muscle is often found when the technique of deep connective tissue massage is used in the abdominal region. This method may free this scar tissue or muscle spasm and usually the stitches do not return, unless some other biomechanical reason exists. A tight and shortened iliopsoas, or fibrous tissue of the abdominal muscle post-natally, are often common precursors to stitches.

Stitches of the shoulder are not so clearly understood. It is of interest to the author that athletes with shoulder stitches are usually kyphotic or have tight pectoral muscles. This type of posture severely overloads the upper thoracic spine. Nerves from this region refer to the anterior chest wall and with postural corrective exercises, mobilisation and stretching of pectorals, the problem is usually relieved. Therefore, it does seem as if this could be a possible mechanism for this type of shoulder complaint.

How do I know when I can return to full sporting activity and what precautions I can take to prevent trauma recurring?

Your specialist or therapist is the person to answer this if you were badly injured but if you have been treating yourself the following points may help you decide.

- Be sure not to return to sport too soon following trauma. Even though there is no pain, an area is healing long after this.

- Ligaments take 2–6 weeks to heal completely.
- Mild muscle strains take 2–14 days to heal, but more severe strains can take 3–6 weeks.
- Cartilage trauma takes 3–6 weeks and if torn may need to be operated on (for instance, the knee). Procedures such as arthroscopy mean rapid recovery and return to sport if a cartilage is the only damage in the knee (when the ligament is not damaged as well).
- Bone fractures take 2–3 months or longer to heal.
- Stress fractures take a minimum of 4–6 weeks before full weight-bearing activities should be resumed.
- Tendonitis, musculoligamentous strains and contusions (from direct trauma impact) are variable in how long they take to heal. They are dependent on the acuteness, extent and mechanism of the injury, and the time that the area has been traumatised prior to treatment. Overuse injuries may need considerable rest or a change in training methods compared with acute injuries where all treatment is aimed at return to sport as soon as it is safe to do so.
- Children's muscle and tendon injuries heal more quickly than adults', but if damage to the bony growth plates has occurred (such as in the knee), rest from sports may be needed for 2–3 months. Seeking advice in the early stages, when a child complains of pain, can prevent these problems.

The following precautions should be taken to minimise the risk of recurrence of a problem.

- Use taping or a guard to support the injured area.
- Try to identify the demands and skills of the sport you are returning to. Consider your current level of fitness; is it adequate? Does your sport require agility skills, flexibility, or specific strength? Reassess technique regularly and play practice matches prior to competition sport. Consult a sports specialist for further advice regarding your training programme if you are returning to sport from having an overuse problem.

Checklist

- Self-help for soft tissue trauma is to use the RICE(D) principle. R = Rest, I = Ice, C = Compression, E = Elevation, D = Diagnosis.
- If the problem does not settle or show signs of improvement within 24–48 hours post-injury, consult a specialist.
- For long term care of an injury, do not return too soon to sport and prepare your body in all aspects of your sport prior to returning to play.

While you are injured, try to participate in some other form of fitness. If you cannot run, swim. If you cannot swim, cycle. If you cannot cycle, then walk. If you are unable to undertake any of these activities because of your pain, you can still stretch regularly to maintain muscle flexibility and tone.

10 — WHO CAN HELP?

There are so many professionals offering cures and remedies for both acute and chronic ailments that it is very difficult to know where to turn. Traditionally, we have turned to our own doctor for medical advice, but with the wide skills required from our local general practitioner he cannot be a specialist in all areas. If you are actively involved in sport, it is best to consult a doctor who specialises in sports injuries. If he is unable to assist you he will refer you to either a specialist in sports injuries, such as a physiotherapist, or to an orthopaedic surgeon. The latter specialises in musculoskeletal disorders, and acts as a diagnostic physician as well as being a skilled surgeon.

An x-ray may be recommended by your local doctor and a radiographer will take the pictures. A radiologist will analyse and write a report on the x-rays. Normal x-rays only show up bone and joint and some visceral related problems, but ligament laxity can be diagnosed if the correct views are shown. Normal cartilage and muscle tissue do not show up on the x-ray. Sometimes soft tissue swelling will show up.

Special investigations called Isotope bone scans and C.A.T. (Computerised Axial Tomography) provide much more detail of bone, soft tissue and bone disorders. Stress fractures are not readily detected on normal x-ray until three to four weeks post-fracture. At this stage new bone formation is able to be detected. These types of fractures (they usually occur in the feet or shins) may be detected by bone scan from as soon as they occur. C.A.T. scans are often used for detecting disc protrusions or prolapses, or nerve impingement problems in the spine.

More recently, a scan called Magnetic Resonance Imaging (M.R.I.) is being used. This is a highly sophisticated investigation which is almost 100 times more accurate than other forms of radiography in depicting soft tissue, bony disc and even cartilage disorders. This has markedly improved the accuracy of clinical diagnosis, particularly where surgery for a musculoskeletal condition is being considered.

There are many other specialists beside the traditional ones. Because of their more recent popularity some of these are labelled 'alternative'. Ironically many of the skills and 'medications' offered by these specialists derive their roots from methods used many years before western medicine developed. Naturopathy and homeopathy are but two of these. Unfortunately many of the substances prescribed by these specialists have not been subjected to the scientific investigation that drugs used in western medicine are put through before being sold by

SELF-HELP CARE

We may feel an ache or a pain somewhere but unless it is debilitating we tend to think it will go away. Weeks and often months later we finally consult someone and then not only does the original problem require treatment but also the compensations, that is, how the body has learnt to survive with the pain. Remember pain is the body's way of telling us something is wrong.

While it is difficult to be black and white about when to seek advice and when to help a problem yourself, always try to use common sense. A useful rule of thumb is that if a pain or ache doesn't settle or show signs of improving within 24–48 hours, seek advice.

Hopefully some of the people you can turn to for professional advice should also be clearer now. Be sure though to be objective about the therapy or treatment you are receiving. If you don't understand why something is being done to you, ask and question why. If you are receiving treatment for an acute injury from a hands-on specialist, that is someone that does massage or manipulation as opposed to someone who uses indirect techniques such as electrotherapy, subscribed exercise, medication or herbal remedies, you should start to see a change or signs of improvement in your condition after three visits. If you don't, you may need to consult a different specialist. Chronic problems of course will take longer but results in the first few visits should be visible. Even being worse after your initial visit may be a sign that your condition is improving, but you obviously shouldn't stay this way!

Sometimes it is difficult to find someone who can clearly define and explain your problem, but remember, having a label for your pain often doesn't help it go away. So don't keep hunting for a definitive label. While this is extremely important in many instances, be sure to take some positive action yourself. Try to be involved with your treatment and helping yourself, particularly if the pain is of musculoskeletal origin. While 'rest' has an important place in the healing process, consider doing some other form of activity if you have been told this is advisable.

Lastly, if your pain persists or your poor posture doesn't seem to be changing, you may need to look beyond your body and its muscles. John Harrison wrote a whole book on pain and disease titled *Love Your Disease* (1984) and claims often we need it! So ask yourself: Do I need my pain or poor posture, and if so, why? Brugh Joy wrote 'disease (and pain) is simply doing for us what we ourselves refuse to do' (*Joy's Way,* 1979), or at least refuse to acknowledge. It certainly is interesting that we sprain our ankle, hurt our back or break a leg always at the worst possible time. What is this telling us — to slow down maybe? Why does an athlete strain a muscle just before a top event? Was it purely an accident related to training or simply a mishap? Certainly question yourself if this is always happening to you!

CHECKLIST

Doctors, orthopedic surgeons, physiotherapists, radiologists and podiatrists have been traditionally seen as the specialists of musculoskeletal disorders.

Natural therapies such as those used by chiropractors, osteopaths, naturopaths/homeopaths, acupuncturists and masseurs are now widely accepted by both the community and health professionals.

When considering who to consult, remain objective and questioning, and if you are not seeing visible results consider changing your practitioner.

THE LAST WORD ON MUSCLES

Do you feel you understand your body a little better now? There's no reason why we should not understand how our bodies function. Unfortunately, from a young age we are conditioned to ignore pain. The longer we cope with it, the greater the heroes we are for doing so. It is indeed a strange attitude.

Ida Rolf, in her book on postural and structural integration, quotes the philosopher Norbert Weiner: 'We are not stuff that abides, but patterns that perpetuate themselves'. That is, we cannot avoid the daily stresses on our bodies from emotions, environment, work and so on. However, if we overreact to them, we become walking 'biological concrete', cemented together with tight muscles creating joint stiffness and poor posture. This in turn may cause pain.

Hopefully, *The Muscle Fitness Book* has dispelled the age-old myth that pain is a natural part of getting old. It does not matter what your age, you can neither be too young nor too old to improve the efficiency of your body. Regular stretching, strengthening, maintaining ideal posture, keeping aerobically fit and sound nutrition are the keys to good health. As you become fitter you will be surprised how much more energy you have each day to carry out your daily chores. Once you are fully involved in your fitness programme you will wonder how you ever lived without it.

Furthermore, no matter what level of sport you play, you will be pleasantly surprised at the extra ease with which you are able to play it, when you incorporate some of the exercises described in this book as part of your warm-up or cool down. By analysing your posture and being aware of the areas most vulnerable to injury in your activity, you will also not need to race from one practitioner to another, in an attempt to find someone who will give you advice other than 'rest' if you do get an injury.

If you do not currently engage in regular sport, *The Muscle Fitness Book* has hopefully convinced you of the merits of doing so. It is never too late to start some form of fitness. Starting with the daily programmes, if you take care as you do each exercise you will be surprised how quickly your muscles start to tone, you improve your flexibility, and most important of all, you will start to feel more positive about yourself. If you have an injury at present which you believe prevents you from exercising, question the advice you have received, particularly if it is from a well-meaning friend. Become more objective about whom you listen to. Reconsider the suitability of your advice. If rest seems unnecessarily advised, where possible seek a second opinion. Don't give up trying to find some way, any possible way, that you may be able to help yourself.

Remember, if you look at someone (child or adult) and see that they look tired, fatigued or appear to be collapsing into gravity (sadly, this is most of us), then keep in mind the key words: if you can predict, you can prevent. Do not let the chain reaction of injury, sedentary lifestyle or excessive exercise damage your muscles or posture in the long term.

If you have children, after reading *The Muscle Fitness Book*, you should now be able to observe them as they are growing and be aware of the importance of early intervention to prevent problems in later years. If they are complaining of pain in their muscles or joints — be aware — it just may be real!

Finally, just remember, your body really doesn't like pain, it wants to feel well and free — what better incentive to keeping your muscles well than this? Happy exercising — keep thinking tall and positive, but most importantly of all, keep having lots of fun!

GLOSSARY

Acromioclavicular joint — the bony prominence on the top of the shoulder, where the clavicle (collar bone) joins the scapula.

Actin — the thinner protein filament in the myofibril which comprise skeletal muscle.

Active range of movement — how far an individual can move a particular part of their body, for example, lifting the arm above the head.

Adaptive shortening — the shortening that occurs over a period of time in a muscle when it is not used through its full range. For example, if the pectoralis major is not used through its full range, adaptive shortening may occur causing round shoulders.

Aerobic exercise — exercise which utilises oxygen from the air, to provide the energy required for exercising, for example, jogging and swimming.

Agonist — the muscle which is contracting.

Alexander technique — a method taught to assist postural correction, designed by Mathias Alexander in the early 1900s.

Anabolic steroid — a drug taken to improve athletic performance. It assists muscle bulking, and a competitive attitude is often developed. **Many negative side-effects.**

Anaerobic exercise — exercise which does not depend on oxygen for its energy. There are two systems that may be used to produce the energy required for this type of exercise: the lactate or the phospate system.

Analgesic effect — a numbing effect exerted in an area, for example, with ice on muscle tissue.

Antagonist — the muscle which relaxes and lengthens when the opposing muscle, the agonist, is contracting, the two working together to effect movement from a joint.

Arteriole — similiar structure to arteries, but much smaller. Most nerve input to the blood vessels goes to the arterioles which is why vasoconstriction and vasodilation are special functions of the arterioles.

Artery — strong blood vessel which is rather elastic in structure. Arteries transport oxygen-rich blood away from the heart.

Arthroscopy — a surgical procedure performed using a scope inserted via a large needle, as opposed to cutting open an area to operate. Removal of torn cartilage of the knee is commonly performed by this technique.

Axillary region — the armpit.

Ball and socket joint — one bony surface is concave and the other convex, which allows a wide range of movement. For example, the shoulder and the hip joint.

Ballistic stretching — fast, dynamic stretching. In fitness classes, this refers to a double bounce on a muscle at the end of its range. It can be potentially hazardous.

Basal metabolic rate — the rate at which the body uses energy while at rest to sustain vital bodily functions.

Biomechanical efficiency — how effectively the body operates with absolute minimal stress on specific joints. For example, being 'pigeon-toed' is biomechanically inefficient when jogging.

Bipedal gait — walking on two limbs only, for example, human beings.

Body contact sport — where physical contact between individual players in a sport is made, for example, football.

Bunion — a callous thickening usually found in the feet. Bunions develop where joints are being loaded abnormally. That is, the individual may be biomechanically inefficient.

Cardiac muscle — muscle surrounding and comprising the heart.

Cardiopulmonary system — the cardiovascular and the respiratory systems.

Cardiovascular system — the heart and the blood vessels.

Carotid arterial pulse — the pulse of the carotid artery, which can be felt at the side and slightly anterior in the neck.

Cartilage — substance protecting the bony surfaces of articulating surfaces of joints.

Cartilaginous disc — the spine is made up of these discs which provide support, as well as having shock-absorbing qualities. Located between each vertebra in the spine.

Cell — the most basic unit of the body.

Cerebrospinal fluid — the fluid which protects and surrounds the brain and the spinal cord.

Cervical vertebrae — the seven vertebrae in the neck.

Concentric contraction — when a muscle shortens as it contracts. Also called a *positive contraction.*

Conditioning phase — the period when an individual commences or resumes a fitness programme, and the heart and lungs subsequently become more efficient. This is called the conditioning phase of an exercise programme.

Connective tissue — the non-contractile white fibrous tissue which separates and supports muscles and all other visceral structures.

Counter-irritant effect — occurs when another stimulus is used to override a specific pain, as when local heat rubs create a warming effect and can reduce pain.

Craniosacral system — the physiological system in the human body which provides the environment in which the brain and spinal cord develop and function. Until the early 1900s this system was relatively unknown. All animals who have a brain and spinal cord (all vertebrates) possess a craniosacral system.

Deep connective tissue massage — a form of massage that works with not only the contractile, but also the non-contractile, components of the myofascial unit. The predominant aim of this type of massage is to influence the fascia.

Disc protrusions — occur when a portion of the disc separating each vertebrae protrudes or bulges beyond the limits of the spinal canal.

Dynamic stretching — stretches which involve motion through a wide range at relatively fast speeds. For instance, kicking the leg high to meet an outstretched hand would be dynamic stretching of the hamstring muscle group.

Dysfunction — when a muscle is not being used in its anatomically correct range, (for example, a shortened pectoralis major muscle causing round shoulders would be in a state of dysfunction).

Eccentric contraction — occurs when a muscle is lengthening. Also called a *negative contraction*. For example, the biceps, while lowering a weight in the hand from a flexed elbow position, are used eccentrically.

Electrotherapy — treatment methods which use electrical equipment to promote or speed up the rate of healing in damaged tissue.

End range — the end point, or how far, a joint can be taken, either by the individual or by a therapist.

Epicondyle — the bony protruberances located on the distal end both medially and laterally on the humerus.

Epicondylitis — an inflammation of the epicondyle. For example, 'tennis elbow' is often a form of epicondylitis.

Epiphyseal plate — or 'growth plate', these are found in growing bone.

Ergometer — a piece of equipment used for fitness testing. For example, a bicycle or treadmill.

Explosive isometric contraction — when an isometric contraction is commenced very suddenly, for example, an arm wrestle. This can be damaging to the muscle.

Extensor — the muscles which straighten a joint after it has been flexed. For example, the extensors of the back bring us back to the standing position when they contract, after we have bent forward touching our toes.

Fascia — a form of connective tissue. It separates, supports and interconnects muscles, organs and bones. It surrounds muscles and separates them and is also found around each myofibril.

Fascial work — a massage technique where the aim is to free the fascia which surrounds the muscle belly, as well as release any fascial adhesions it may have with its neighbouring muscles. A form of deep connective tissue massage.

Fast-twitch fibre — these are found in skeletal muscle. They are characterised by a quick response to stimulation. Physiologically, they have a high capability for anaerobic metabolism. Sprinting activities utilise predominately fast-twitch fibres.

Feldenkrais method — a method of working with the body devised by Mosh Feldenkrais. Its main goal is to deprogramme poor postural and muscular habits and reprogramme new patterns by gentle awareness through movement exercises. A skilled Feldenkrais practitioner can teach the individual these movements.

Femoral angle — in the hip, the femoral angle of inclination is formed by the neck and shaft of the femur. It is normally 125 degrees, but varies in inverse proportion to the development of the width and stature of the pelvis. For example, females have a greater femoral angle compared with males because of their inherently broader pelvis.

Femoral anteversion — internal rotation of the femur.

Femoral retroversion — external rotation of the femur.

Femoral torsion — the inward or outward curve of the femur in relation to the hip.

Fibrositis — occurs when tension or an overload of muscle becomes chronic and an increase in fibrin tissue results. Blood supply to this area becomes impeded and inflammation within the muscle may occur.

Fixator — the muscle required to fix or stabilise a joint while muscles located peripherally are working more actively through their range. For example, exercising the biceps by bending the elbows while the arms are held in horizontal abduction. Here the deltoid would be the fixator.

Flat feet — no visible arch is apparent when an individual is standing, that is, when the entire sole of the foot touches the ground. Often referred to as overpronation.

Gait cycle — patterns of walking. The gait cycle refers inclusively to the swing and stance phase of the gait.

Gastrocnemius — the largest muscle below the knee, usually called the *calf muscle*. When it contracts, it points the foot. This is called *plantaflexion*.

Gastrointestinal system — all organs and parts of the system which utilise, digest and absorb food and excrete waste products.

Genu recurvatum — hyperextension of the knees, often called swayback knees. Usually occurs because of hypermobility.

Glenohumeral joint — the shoulder joint, a ball and socket joint.

Gross movement — the main movement performed actively by an individual when exercising. For example, picking up an object off a table requires gross movement at the shoulder, but finer movements of the fingers.

Growth plate — occurs when new bone is laid down to permit growth in a bone, in the epiphysis of the bone.

Harvard step test — a very basic test which utilises a step as an ergometer to test an individual's level of fitness.

Hellerwork — a technique of bodywork based on the works of Joseph Heller. It is a system of working with muscle and fascia (called neuro-myofascial re-education) to improve posture and works with the emotional tensions we carry in our body.

Hinge joint — any joint which permits minimal rotation, only flexion and extension. Open and close in a similar way to a door hinge: elbows, knees and toes.

Histamine — a chemical released by the body in response to pain and inflammation, and post-exercise.

Hypermobility — when an individual is overly flexible. Usually this extra flexibility is due to extra length in the ligaments and an increased passive range of movement is noted. It is often incorrectly labelled 'double-jointed'.

Hypertrophy — when there is an increase in the bulk or size of muscle.

Hypothalamic response — the means by which the body regulates temperature is controlled by the hypothalmus, a part of the brain.

Inner range — working a joint while the agonists are contracted and working in a very small range. For example, raising the thigh while side lying, only lifting the leg 10 to 15 degrees, would be strengthening the hip abductors in their inner range.

Insertion — where a muscle attaches to bone. Usually refers to the most distal point of attachment.

Intervertebral joint — the joint between each of the vertebrae of the spine.

Involuntary movement — when a muscle contracts suddenly without the individual thinking about contracting it. For example, this occurs in the arm when something very hot is touched. This is an involuntary movement.

Ischaemia — excessive blood pooling that occurs in muscle while exercising.

Isometric contraction — when a change in tension occurs in a muscle, but the length of the muscle stays virtually the same. For example, an isometric contraction occurs in the arm muscles during an arm wrestle.

Juvenile arthritis — inflammation of the joints in a child or a teenager.

Kinesiology — the study of movement and motion.

Kinetic system — any system where each part of it is in some way influenced when changes occur in other parts of the system. The body is often called a kinetic system.

Lactic acid — the waste product formed when glycogen (muscle energy or fuel) is only partially broken down in the absence of oxygen. Lactic acid is produced with anaerobic activity, but is removed almost entirely from the muscles and blood within the 45 to 60 minutes after the exercise is completed. It is *not* responsible for post-exercise soreness as is commonly thought.

Ligament — a relatively inelastic fibrous band which connects bones and thus provides joint stability. Once overstrained or over-stretched, they often never return to their original shape or strength.

Lumbar roll — a small, long and round cushion which can be used in the small of the back to retain the lumbar curve (lordosis) when sitting.

Lymph node — small nodules found throughout the body. Accumulations are found in the armpit and in the groin. They are part of the lymphatic system.

Lymphatic system — the system which is primarily responsible for fighting infection in the body. It comprises lymph capillaries and lymph vessels, and these provide a pathway whereby tissue fluid is returned to the blood stream.

Magnetic resonating investigation — a specialised radiological technique which is able to show damage to structures such as cartilage and disc, previously not detectable by usual x-ray techniques.

Manipulation — physical techniques which influence joints or muscle with the hands. Specific joint manipulation refers to high velocity adjustments, performed by a specialised manipulative practitioner, where the patient is not able to control the movement executed on a specific joint.

Maximum heart rate — (MHR) the highest heart rate an individual will achieve. A general formula to calculate the approximate MHR is to subtract the individual's age from 220.

Medial epicondyle — the bony protruberance on the medial aspect of the elbow. Often this is the problem area for 'golfer's elbow'.

Mobilisation — controlled graded movements, used by skilled health practitioners, to directly influence and improve the passive joint range of movement of a joint.

Motor function — the motor nervous system, as opposed to the sensory nervous system. Motor function refers more specifically to musculoskeletal movement.

Motor nerve — these are nerves which supply muscle. When stimulated either voluntarily, involuntarily, or electrically, a muscle contraction will result.

Multipennate — one of the muscle shapes. In this type of muscle, fibres run in many different directions. The deltoid is an example of a multipennate muscle.

Muscle belly — the fleshy bulk of a muscle in the middle of the tendinous insertions on either end.

Muscle tone — the 'tautness' or 'firmness' of a muscle when the body is at rest. Body builders and fit individuals have excellent muscle tone, unfit individuals do not.

Muscles — these comprise 40 per cent of the body's mass. There are three different types of muscle, smooth, cardiac and striated. The major role of skeletal muscles is to move bones.

Musculoligamentous — refers collectively to both the muscles and the ligaments which surround and support a joint.

Musculoskeletal system — the skeleton and its associated bones, the ligaments, tendons, and the muscles.

Myofascial unit — a muscle and the fascia which directly surrounds it.

Myofibril — the component of a muscle cell that distinguishes it from all other cells. Skeletal muscle is composed of thousands of myofibrils bound together by connective tissue and contained in a fluid called sarcoplasm.

Myosin — a myofibril contains two basic protein filaments: the thicker one is called myosin, the thinner actin.

Nerve — part of the nervous system, they carry the electrical impulses from the brain via the spinal cord. Permit movement of muscle or sensation in all body parts.

Nerve impingement — when a nerve is trapped mechanically by bony structures or by muscle, within the body. When nerves are impinged in the neck or lower back, pain may radiate peripherally to either the arm or the leg.

Nervous system — comprises the brain, spinal cord and all nerves in the body.

Non-contractile — the portion of the muscle where motor nerves do not go and where no contraction occurs. Connective tissue is part of the non-contractile component of muscle.

Origin — the point of origin of a muscle off the bone.

Orthotics — devices which are used inside shoes to correct faulty foot biomechanics. For example, orthotics may be needed to correct 'flat-feet'.

Osteoarthritis — a condition with degeneration of articulating joint surfaces.

Osteoporosis — thinning of the matrix of bones making them soft and brittle.

Passive range of movement — how far a skilled therapist can move (that is, mobilise or manipulate) a joint. The passive range of movement is not able to be performed by individuals themselves.

Patello-femoral — the region under the patella (knee cap) which rides over the femur. This is usually the affected area in 'runner's knee'.

Peripheral joint — joints not directly attached to the trunk or torso. Elbow, knee, etc. are examples of peripheral joints.

Pexiplave — a hard synthetic surface which is used on a tennis court. It is called an all-weather surface as it permits seepage of water through it if it rains.

Phasic muscle — muscles which are used (that is, 'electrically' activated) predominately when we move.

Physiotherapist — a skilled health practitioner, who treats a wide range of health disorders by using physical assistance of the hands and electrotherapeutic modalities, exercise, etc.

Piriformis — a muscle located deep in the buttocks. If it is in spasm, the sciatic nerve which usually passes through its bulk is compressed. This may be called *sciatica*.

Pituitary cortex — a portion of the brain which comprises the pituitary gland. This gland secretes hormones which influence many of the endocrine glands of the body.

Pivot joint — occur where a ring of bone rotates around a bony prominence on another bone. An example is the first cervical vertebra at the base of the skull which rotates around the second cervical vertebra.

Plantar fascitis — inflammation of the plantafascia, a strong fibrous strip of connective tissue which assists with the support of the arch of the foot.

Plantar wart — often found in the heel or the ball of the foot, they form and grow underneath the skin. If painful, surgical removal is required.

Plyometrics — a form of muscle training which comprises a concentric contraction, followed suddenly by an eccentric contraction. Basketballers use this form of training to improve the effectiveness of their jumping.

PNF stretching — proprioceptive neuromuscular facilitation. One of the most effective ways to elongate a muscle, it involves contracting a muscle isometrically against an immovable object for 6 to 10 second; then relaxing the muscle, taking it into a new lengthened position, then repeating this procedure 2 to 3 times. Partner stretching is helpful to do PNF work.

Podiatrist — a health practitioner who specialises in the care of feet, and who is able to asses and treat mechanical foot disorders.

Postural grid-plate — a grid which permits assessment of posture by measuring deviation from the midline (using a plumball). Photos may record postural deviations.

Postural muscles — the muscles which are still 'electrically' active when we are standing, sitting or lying down. They are still used when we move, but continue to be active when we stop. Phasic muscles do not.

Prolapse — when there is a protrusion of the disc in the intervertebral space. It may protrude into the spinal canal and aggravate nerve structures. This can be extremely painful.

Protoplasm — the jelly-like substance of the cell, where complex biochemical changes occur, forming the processes of life.

Prime mover — the major muscle contracting in any particular movement.

Physical work capacity (PWC) 170 — a method of establishing an individual's level of fitness.

Range — how far a muscle can move a joint.

Range of movement stretching — this involves taking a muscle through the range it is about to be worked in. For example, range of movement stretching is used in aquarobics while in the water by swinging the leg forwards and backwards from the hip to stretch the hamstrings.

Rebounder — a mini-trampoline used for fitness purposes.

Relaxin — a hormone released during pregnancy which affects the ligaments of the pelvis, hips and lower back. These ligaments become softened due to the effect of this hormone.

Resisted exercise machines — machines used in weight-training to provide resistance to a muscle to enable it to be strengthened.

Respiratory system — the lungs and air passages.

Resting heart rate — an individual's heart rate when at rest. This can be assessed by taking the pulse of a resting individual.

Rheumatoid arthritis — a systemic disease which causes stiffness and immobility of joints.

Rolfing — a form of deep tissue work, often called postural and structural integration, developed by Ida Rolf. The intent is to restore postural and muscular imbalance and to release emotional tensions 'stored' in our muscles.

Sacroiliac joint — the joint where the sacrum (the base of the spine) joins the hip bone (the ilium).

Sarcoplasm — the fluid in which the myofibrils of the skeletal muscle and its associated connective tissue is found.

Sciatic nerve — the largest nerve in the body. It originates from the spine at the level of the lumbar and sacral vertebra. It then runs through the buttock and branches as it tranverses down the posterior aspect of the leg.

Shoulder girdle — the shoulder, neck, upper spine and rib cage.

Skeletal muscle — also called striated muscle. It is responsible for voluntary movement of the body.

Sliding joint — joints that move from side to side and up and down. They can also rotate but not as freely as a ball and socket joint. Examples are the wrist and ankle joints. There are also known as ellipsoid joints.

Slow-twitch fibre — fibres located in skeletal muscle that contract more slowly than fast-twitch fibres. They are utilised most in endurance activities which depend almost entirely on the energy generated by aerobic metabolism.

Smooth muscle — the type of muscle found in the arteries and stomach. It is to a large extent under involuntary control.

Somatotype — an individuals body shape. There are three basic shapes; (a) ectomorph: tall and thin; (b) mesomorph: average height and muscular; (c) endomorph: short and plump. Most of us have characteristics of one or more of these body types.

Spinal canal — where the spinal cord runs down through the spine through each vertebra.

Stance phase — the times when the foot is planted on the ground in a normal gait cycle.

Static stretching — occurs when a muscle is put on stretch (that is, taken to the end of its range) held from 6 to 30 seconds, even longer, then when one relaxes, a new length in the muscle can be achieved. This is repeated 2 to 3 times at a minimum.

Stone bruise — when bruising occurs under the top layer of the skin. This most commonly occurs in the heels.

Strength training — when muscle training is done using the resistance provided by weights.

Stretch-reflex — a protective reflex which prevents overstretching of a muscle. For example, if the head drops forward while someone is sitting, and they doze off to sleep, the stretch reflex is activated in the neck extensors which causes them to contract suddenly. This protects the neck in this instance from overstretching.

Sublux — when a joint slides slightly out of its stable position. This is not the same as dislocation, which is when a bone comes entirely out of its position. A subluxing joint usually indicates overlengthened and overstretched ligaments, either due to trauma or to excessive hypermobility.

Sub-maximal test — a method of testing fitness where an individual is not stressed to their maximum heart rate, but figures are extrapolated from the sub-maximal test to identify how well the athlete or person will cope, when they are exercising at a maximal level.

Substance p — refers to a substance produced in the body during exercise, which stimulates nerve endings causing muscle spasm, which in turn causes muscle pain.

Synergist — a synergist assists the agonist in prime movement of a body part.

Tai Chi — a series of movement and awareness exercises developed in the Eastern Countries. It is claimed to harmonise body forces and return them to normal.

Tendon — where a muscle approaches its attachment site with a bone, the contractile elements of that muscle end, and connective tissue known as tendons form the attachment.

Testosterone — the male hormone, though females do have some present in their bodies. It is responsible for male characteristics, such as a deepened voice, growth of hair on the chest, etc.

Tibial torsion — normally the tibia is externally twisted about 12 degrees along its length. This is called tibial torsion. Excessive external tibial torsion (that is, greater than 20 degrees) may result in patello-femoral and other knee disorders.

Tissue — groups of cells combined together to perform a similar function.

Torsion — the rotational deviation that occurs in long bones. Mostly used in reference to the weight-bearing bones such as the femur and tibia.

Trager therapy — a form of bodywork expounded by Milton Trager. An approach that works with the psychophysical. It aims to improve the way an individual moves and functions.

Trunk muscle — muscles which influence the spine and its associated structures, for example, the rib cage, the vertebrae, etc.

Unipennate — the shape of a muscle where all fibres run in one and the same direction.

Vasoconstriction — when blood vessels (the arterioles) become smaller. This occurs when ice is placed on the body and is under control of the sympathetic nervous system. (part of the automatic nervous system).

Vasodilation — when the blood vessels (the arterioles) become larger. Occurs when heat is applied to the body. It is under the control of the parasympathetic nervous system.

Vein — a blood vessel which returns blood to the heart. They have valves in them to assist the pumping of fluid up the body against gravity.

Vertebrae — the individual bones that comprise the spinal column. There are 24 moveable bones and seven less flexible ones.

Vertebral joints — the joints connecting the vertebrae. Each individual joint has only limited movement. However, when the vertebrae move together, the spine can bend in all directions as well as rotate.

Vertebral level — a specific level in the spine. For example, T12 refers to the 12th vertebral level of the thoracic spine, where the 12th rib attaches.

Video analysis — the use of a video camera to analyse the body, either stationary, moving or in a particular sporting activity.

Viscera — organs in the gastrointestinal system.

Voluntary movement — a movement performed by an individual under their own volition. For example, lifting up a cup off a table involves voluntary movement of the forearm muscles.

GENERAL HEALTH AND FITNESS

Hazeldine, R., *Fitness for Sports* (The Crowood Press, 1988)
Hazeldine, R., *Strength Training for Sport* (The Crowood Press, 1990)

STRETCHES AND EXERCISE MANUALS

Alter, M. J., *Science of Stretching* (Human Kinetics, 1988)
Anderson, B., *Stretching* (Pelham, 1981)
Feldenkrais, M., *Awareness Through Movement* (Harper & Row, 1972)
Ryan, A. J. and Stephens, R. E., *Dance Medicine* (Plumbus Press and The Physician and Sportsmedicine, 1987)

SPORTS MEDICINE AND SCIENCE

Egger, G., *The Sport Drug* (Allen & Unwin, 1982)
Fox, E. L., *Sports Physiology* (W.B. Saunders, 1979)
Grisogono, V., *Sports Injuries: a self-help guide* (Murray, 1984)
Rolf, I., *Rolfing: The Integration of Human Structures* (Harper & Row, 1977)
Roy, S. and Irvin, R., *Sports Medicine* (Prentice Hall, 1983)
Wilmore, J. H., 'Body Composition in Sport and Exercise: Directions for Future Research' (*Medicine and Science in Sport and Exercise*, vol. 13, 1983)
Wirhead, R., *Athletic Ability and the Anatomy of Motion* (Wolfe, 1985)

HOLISTIC HEALTH

Barlow, W., *The Alexander Technique* (Random House, 1973)
Harrison, J., *Love your Disease* (Angus & Robertson, 1984)
Joy, W. B., *Joy's Way* (Tarder, 1979)

INDEX